VALUES IN PSYCHOLOGICAL SCIENCE

In this book, wide-ranging sources are utilized to seek alternatives to the science-value dichotomy and to move beyond unhelpful impasses between qualitative and quantitative methods. It urges new directions of impact for psychology through intra- and interdisciplinary collaboration in order to confront unprecedented global challenges, generate questions, and articulate new possibilities for a sustainable future for humanity. The analysis places the researcher as the principal instrument of any science – an affordance and an ongoing form of demand. Foregrounding "the personal" also emphasizes continuity across arts and sciences, the interfaces of which contain the full range of resources for innovative thinking. The enduring relevance of observation, imaginative sense-making, and perspective-taking to psychology is explored. In emphasizing that "the person" and "the personal" reflect interconnected systems of various levels, the book calls for an appreciation and cultivation of these activities in the psychological scientific community.

Lisa Osbeck is a Professor of Psychology, University of West Georgia, and a Fellow of the Center for Philosophy of Science, University of Pittsburgh, and the American Psychological Association (APA).

Values in Psychological Science

REIMAGINING EPISTEMIC PRIORITIES AT A NEW
FRONTIER

Lisa Osbeck

University of West Georgia

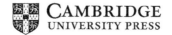

CAMBRIDGE
UNIVERSITY PRESS

CAMBRIDGE
UNIVERSITY PRESS

University Printing House, Cambridge CB2 8BS, United Kingdom

One Liberty Plaza, 20th Floor, New York, NY 10006, USA

477 Williamstown Road, Port Melbourne, VIC 3207, Australia

314–321, 3rd Floor, Plot 3, Splendor Forum, Jasola District Centre, New Delhi – 110025, India

79 Anson Road, #06–04/06, Singapore 079906

Cambridge University Press is part of the University of Cambridge.

It furthers the University's mission by disseminating knowledge in the pursuit of education, learning, and research at the highest international levels of excellence.

www.cambridge.org
Information on this title: www.cambridge.org/9781107134904
DOI: 10.1017/9781316471302

First published 2019

Printed and bound in Great Britain by Clays Ltd, Elcograf S.p.A.

A catalogue record for this publication is available from the British Library.

Library of Congress Cataloging-in-Publication Data
NAMES: Osbeck, Lisa M., 1962– author.
TITLE: Values in psychological science : re-imagining epistemic priorities at a new frontier / Lisa Osbeck.
DESCRIPTION: Cambridge, United Kingdom ; New York, NY : Cambridge University Press, 2019] | Includes bibliographical references.
IDENTIFIERS: LCCN 2018026133 | ISBN 9781107134904 (hbk.)
SUBJECTS: LCSH: Psychology – Study and teaching. | Psychology – Philosophy.
CLASSIFICATION: LCC BF77 .O83 2019 | DDC 150.71–dc23
LC record available at https://lccn.loc.gov/2018026133

ISBN 978-1-107-13490-4 Hardback

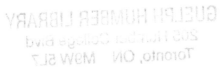

To Kenneth and Ceci, whom I remember singing

CONTENTS

PREFACE

What it comes back to, for the mature mind – granting of course, to begin with, a mind accessible to questions of such an order – is this attaching speculative interest of the matter . . .

The old matter is there, re-accepted, re-tasted, exquisitely re-assimilated and enjoyed – believed in, to be brief, with the same 'old' grateful faith . . .

yet for due testimony, for reassertion of value, perforating as by some strange and fine, some latent and gathered force, a myriad more adequate channels.

Henry James, 2009/1909, p. liii

This book proceeds from the assumption, at once commonplace and radical, that science consists in the creative and responsible acts of persons, and that psychology must do better to try to understand what this implies for its own endeavors. That we never escape ourselves is a pedestrian claim – a truism, even – that we can endorse with little bother. Yet it is precisely the implications of this insight that physicist Bridgman called "the most important problem before us," linked to, but "infinitely more complicated than, the problem of the role of the observer to which quantum theory has devoted so much attention and regards as so fundamental" (1959, pp. 5–6). The present book is modest in its aim, which is to offer only a broad sketch of a framework to recast the "problem" of the "personal" as an affordance for psychology, even as it constitutes an ongoing form of demand. The argument draws from an array of disparate sources, reflecting the peculiar sensibilities, influences, and values of its author.

The "frontier" in question refers to a critical time in human development, a time of exceedingly rapid technological and social transformation and unpredictable global challenges, requiring innovative modes of thinking and new solutions – "frontier science." It is also a reference to a frontier of collaborative potential within psychology and between psychology and other disciplines. After decades of humanistic, constructionist, critical/historical, feminist, phenomenological, discursive, ecological, and other frameworks of critique, new constructive efforts are underway. Psychological humanities (Teo, 2017), indigenous psychology (Sundararajan, 2015), narrative psychology (Josselson & Hopkins, 2015; Kim, 2015; McAdams, 2014; Woolhouse, 2017), and a focus on the psychological "other" (Freeman, 2014) exemplify "movements" at least loosely defined, which begin to generate momentum. They are united in recognition that strictures on psychology and its methods arise from a narrow view of what it means to be scientific, that psychology as both an academic subject and professional pursuit labors under a weighty but sometimes unreflective "scientism" that threatens even to bleed into every domain, overstretching the reach and purpose of science (Williams & Robinson, 2014).

Constructive alternatives emerge from recognition that the impact of critical evaluation of psychology's principal theoretical frameworks and methods remains uncertain. The discipline of psychology as practiced looks less like a robust and constructive pluralism than it does a patchwork of separate, sometimes hostile encampments, with psychologists from different backgrounds and with different convictions tending principally to their respective fires, citing epistemological incompatibility or incommensurability as a reason to avoid collaboration toward a common goal. There are risks in perpetuating too stark a contrast between science and the humanities – risks that include a diminished conception of the embodied, enculturated nature of scientific reasoning and neglect or denial of the sophisticated forms and expressions of "rationality" outside of natural science. In the face of contemporary human challenges and for trials yet to come, we must increasingly look to a new frontier – to the interfaces of sciences and the arts/humanities, in order to understand the deepest interconnections between domains at the level of generative human activity. To the extent that psychology is accessible to questions of such an order, it is in a position for reevaluation and reimagining, for "due testimony and reasserting of value, by myriad more adequate channels."

ACKNOWLEDGMENTS

This manuscript occasionally draws upon material presented or published elsewhere: Osbeck, L. & Nersessian, N. (2017), Epistemic identities in interdisciplinary science, *Perspectives on Science*, 25(2), 226–260; Osbeck, L. & Nersessian, N. J. (2013), Situating distributed cognition, *Philosophical Psychology, Special Issue: Extended Cognition: New Philosophical Perspectives.* 27(1), 82–97. Osbeck, L. & Nersessian, N.J. (2012). The Acting Person in Scientific Practice. In R. Proctor and J. Capaldi (Eds.), *Psychology of Science: Implicit and Explicit Reasoning* (pp. 89–111). New York: Oxford University Press; Osbeck, L. (2005). Method and theoretical psychology. *Theory & Psychology, 15*(1), 5–26. An early version of some of the ideas developed here was presented in the context of the 2016 Arthur W. Staats Lecture for Unifying Psychology, sponsored by the American Psychological Foundation and coordinated by APA Division 1.

I have had the great fortune to work with extraordinary interdisciplinary persons as mentors and collaborators. In order of their appearance in my life, I am especially beholden to Dan Robinson, James Lamiell, Rom Harré, Fathali Moghaddam, Jennifer Clegg, Peter Machamer, Nancy Nersessian, Sanjay Chandrasekharan, Barbara Held, Saulo Araujo, and Giridhari Lal Pandit. I must include Henderikus Stam, who supported my work since I was a graduate student. They all have my heartfelt admiration and gratitude, but they are not responsible for any excesses and omissions in this book or work elsewhere. Thanks also to Ruthellen Josselson, Heidi Levitt, Ron Miller, Michael Stuart, Alan Tjeltveit, and Fred Wertz for especially helpful conversations and resources that relate in at least a broad way to the themes of this work. I am indebted to many additional friends and colleagues in the American Psychological Association Divisions 24 (Society for Theoretical and Philosophical Psychology), 5 (Quantitative and Qualitative

Methods), and 1 (Society for General Psychology). They know, I hope, who they are.

I am grateful to the excellent editorial staff at Cambridge University Press for their support and guidance through all stages of production. I also benefited from the suggestions of four anonymous reviewers on the original proposal for this project, and hope they will not mind some departure from it. Thanks to the Department of Psychology, the College of Social Science, and the VPAA's office at the University of West Georgia for granting me a leave of absence during which to complete the manuscript. Thanks to my students, especially Ram Vivekananda, Garri Hovhannisyan, Dan Eamon Slattery, Suraj Sood, Gary Senecal, India MacWeeney, and Maurice "Dominique" Crossley.

To my family, gratitude abundant and eternal.

1

Introduction

To have a scheme and a view of its dignity is of course congruously to work it out, and the 'amusement' of the chronicle in question – by which, once more, I always mean the gathered cluster of all the kinds of interest, was exactly to see what a consummate application of such sincerities would give.

(Henry James,2009/1909, p. xliv)

The active nature asserts its rights to the end.

(William James,1890, v. 2, p. 314)

This book is intended both as a critique and as a constructive project. It proceeds from conviction that the epistemic priorities of the discipline of psychology are in need of reexamination and reenvisioning in keeping with unprecedented challenges facing humankind, and unforeseeable, even unthinkable, changes ahead of us. It is written at a time when climate change, terrorism, pollution, poverty, genocide, information wars, natural disasters, and nuclear proliferation are daily realities, and when technologies dynamically transform patterns of interaction with extraordinary speed and impact. Although a societal and disciplinary need for moral progress (collective wisdom) is paramount, we also remain in need of groundbreaking conceptual and theoretical resources, resources that require passionate intellectual engagement and imagination in the service of new possibilities. In focusing on epistemic priorities, the project of this book takes inspiration from the idea of "frontier science" – science that seeks new windows of understanding the world – and especially from the suggestion that the generation of resources for creative problem solving is the appropriate epistemic goal for scientific advance, and one conditional to the possibility of a sustainable human future (Pandit and Dosch, 2013).

I am hardly alone in acknowledging a need for new solutions, even new modes of thinking. The rise of interdisciplinary science over the past several decades reflects broad recognition that creative problem solving on the scale required to meet contemporary global challenges of extraordinary complexity requires resources (concepts, models, theories, methods) from more than one discipline or any one branch of inquiry. What is needed, even demanded, in short, is broad and multi-perspectival collaboration to generate a network of flexible, highly adaptable tools. I have attempted here to reimagine the epistemic priorities of psychological science based on conviction that psychology will increasingly find challenge and opportunity for human impact through interdisciplinary participation, through practices focused on the generation of new questions and articulation of new possibilities for a sustainable human future. In developing the ideas, I suggest a set of *activities* in need of greater appreciation and emphasis. The principal thesis I offer is that many of the activities that are "good for psychological science" in the sense of generating resources for problem solving are also activities that are "good for the arts and humanities." The points of commonality in these domains of activity constitute the grounds of possibility for productive collaboration across psychology and between psychology and other disciplines.

PRIORITIZING ACTIVITIES AND PERSONS

In asserting the need for evaluation of psychology's disciplinary priorities, I bracket the question of appropriate or legitimate psychological methods. Activities are more fundamental than methods; they extend beyond psychology into other disciplinary spaces, and beyond research practice into everyday life. The analysis of activities as loci of value stems from adoption of the *acting person* as an analytic focus for understanding science, a focus that finds precedent in philosophy of science (especially Dewey, 1938; Polanyi, 1974/1958), psychological theory (Bergner, 2017; Kelly, 1955; Harré, 1992; Lamiell, 2009; Martin, 2017; Martin & Bickhard, 2013; Rogers, 1963; Smythe, 1998; Wertz, 2016), and ethnographic analysis of scientists in real-world contexts of practice (Osbeck et al., 2011; Osbeck & Nersessian, 2006, 2015, 2017). In keeping with the latter, I consider "the acting person" to be an inherently integrated unit of analysis, one that thus stands as an alternative to accounts of science based principally upon *either* analysis of cognitive mechanism *or* macrosocial processes (Osbeck & Nersessian, 2012).

In calls to prioritize persons in psychology, arguments generally include some version of the claim that the category of "person" as an ontological kind implies attributes such as intentionality, rationality, self-expression, language use, rule following, or individuality/particularity, depending on the philosophical emphasis of the author advocating for the rightful place of persons in psychology and the special conditions for the study of persons (e.g., particular ethical considerations, qualitative analysis enabling participants to express their views and feelings). This book differs from most existing work on persons and psychology in that its emphasis is explicitly on the personhood of the psychological researcher: *the researcher as person*, and the epistemic values that follow from this emphasis. The foregrounding of the personhood of the researcher contrasts with a foregrounding of or emphasis on investigatory procedures and technologies, especially in isolation of the value-laden traditions and contexts in which they are used. The following summary expresses the deep entrenchment of a technique-driven view:

> [G]enerations of students, who, driven by the logic and requirements of a "behavioral science," learned to define scientific problems appreciably in terms of the availability and capability of instruments favored or mandated in their time. The instruments – indeed virtually the entire process of thinking about research – rather quickly took on formidable qualities independent of the persons using them.
>
> (Schatzman & Strauss, 1973, pp. 141–142)

Ethnography has long advocated a contrasting "researcher as instrument" model, one that emphasizes active researcher decision-making and engagement of all activities relating to inquiry – the selection of a research site, the collection of data through interview and observation, the interpretation of data, and decisions about when the research is completed and what should follow. That these decisions incorporate goals, emotion, and historical and cultural situatedness and identity follows as a matter of course. Stressing the fact that the whole person of the researcher is engaged in the research process is, indeed, central to what ethnography means – "it has always meant the attempt to understand another life world using the self – as much of it as possible – as the instrument of knowing" (Ortner, 1995, p. 173). But the claim that the researcher is the instrument for ethnographic investigation can tempt unfortunate contrast with other forms of behavioral research, suggesting that they do not involve whole person activity. Such a suggestion encourages a view that procedures for the collection and analysis of, for example, standardized questionnaire responses are somehow independent of the qualities, motivations, purposes, and interpretive perspective of the researcher by whom such tools are used.

On the most fundamental level, for any method and any empirical project, the empirical instrument includes the researcher, who actively selects and analyzes data for any purpose at hand, selects and employs a set of analytic strategies, creatively participates in generating models, and draws implications from the analysis. That is, the "researcher as instrument" model is applicable to any method of data collection and any form of analysis, despite the different kinds of questions the research addresses and great differences in the degree of interpretive latitude accompanying the use of, for example, narrative vs. multivariate analysis (Osbeck & Nersessian, 2015).

To foreground the researcher as instrument is to emphasize the "acting person" in science, including all forms of psychological science. Importantly, because persons always act within normatively structured contexts of practice that give meaning to their acts, actions are always transactions within systems. Thus to foreground persons does not signal a return to an isolated individualism, but it enables us to consider the particularity of the researcher, the manifest ways in which a unique embodiment and personal history contribute to the complex amalgamation of science practice. As argued elsewhere, wholly cognitive or social accounts are sufficient, and empirical studies of science have long suffered from an "integration problem" (Longino, 2002; Nersessian, 2005). The acting person is an inherently integrated unit of analysis, an integration of social and cognitive processes as well as "something else" not reducible to these categories – a singular configuration of affect, aspirations, interests, and style that inevitably leave their mark (Osbeck et al., 2011), and that contribute to the possibility of scientific achievement (Polanyi, 1974/1958).

One might reasonably substitute "subjectivity" here for "persons" with little loss of meaning, and other authors have found "subjectivity" a more suitable name for the aspect or dimension of science to which we are pointing (e.g., Mahoney, 2004/1976; Mitroff, 1974). The suitability of "subject" and "subjectivity" is found at least in part in the implied contrast with "object" and "objectivity." My own preference for "person" is rooted in its close conceptual relation to the idea of activity, or specifically, active intelligence, itself traceable in at least analogous form to Aristotle, revived by Dewey (1910, 1938), and featured in "enactivist" frameworks in cognitive science that emphasize the inseparability of "activity" from embodiment, coordination with other agents, and resonant attunement with the environment (e.g., Hutto & Myin, 2017; Menary, 2007; Varela, Thompson, & Rosch, 2017).

Long prior to the enactivist tradition, and in a different corner of scholarship, the theological/philosophical tradition of "personalism" offered an inherently integrated unit of analysis in the concept of "person." Personalism, the philosophical system to which "person" is central, "gives *equal recognition* to both the *pluralistic and monistic* aspects of experience" and "finds in the conscious unity, identity, and free activity of the personality the key to the nature of reality and the solution to the ultimate problems of psychology" (Knudson, *Philosophy of Personalism*, quoted by Muelder, 1998). Although the roots of personalism have been traced at least to the fourth century AD, its modern instantiation and appearance as a "system" (an "ism") are attributable to various points of origin. An American version dates to the late nineteenth century through Borden P. Bowne and colleagues at Boston University.[1] Within this framework, "person" is a metaphysical concept, indeed, a "metaphysical primary" (Brightman, 1943), the "double source" of which is both the Greek *hypostasis* and the Latin *persona* (Muelder, 1998, p. xi). The former implies an underlying reality, essence, or substance – an embodiment, we might say; the latter the "actor's mask"– the face shown or the role(s) one plays in relation to myriad others. The idea of social connectedness and the inherent dignity and worth of all persons so connected are important and necessary implications of the metaphysical assumptions. Consequently, ethical considerations are rarely far from any formulation of the features of "person."[2] Thus to foreground persons in psychology is to foreground values, epistemic, aesthetic, moral, and social in kind.

Similarly, the concept of person is closely tied to the idea of activity, or specifically, active intelligence. Personalism established the active, comparing, reducing, and synthesizing intellect as central to the means by which all knowledge is possible, including knowledge we classify as the conceptual basis of any science. Without the integrating activity of persons, there is no scientific advance, but neither is there experience of any kind. Reasoning as an integrated act of persons "does not stand as an intellectual opponent or alternative to the nonrational or irrational givens in human experience, but reason's work is to relate experience of all kinds to one

---

[1] The term "personalism" for the same system of thought followed the publication of Renouvier's *Le Personalisme* in 1903 (Muelder, 1998).

[2] Dr. Martin Luther King, Jr. is considered a fourth-generation personalist in his theological pedigree, with his contributions to the cause of social justice rooted in the metaphysics of personalism (Burrow, 1999).

another coherently and synoptically with modes of analysis, hypothesis, and verification appropriate to each and to the whole:" (Muelder, 1998, p. xiii). These are modes of activity. In turn, "empirically coherent interpretation" serves as a "guide to creative living" (Buford, 2006, p. 214). Thus in turn it triggers the question of what kinds of activities constitute epistemic priorities, such that they are to be valued, encouraged, and cultivated at the level of the psychological community, including in our educative practices.

INSPIRATION, PRECAUTIONS, AND PLAN

Framed as a reimagining of priorities, this book must be owned as a project that is theoretical and principally speculative. However, it is inspired by experience with and reflection on actual practices of communities of scientists engaged in groundbreaking, frontier research. I had the good fortune to collaborate in investigating scientific practice "in the wild" with the *Cognition and Learning in Interdisciplinary Learning Cultures* group led by Nancy Nersessian, and with the collaboration of a team of researchers with a diverse range of disciplinary backgrounds that included Kareen Malone, Nancy Nersessian, Elke Kurz-Milke, and Sanjay Chandrasekharen.[3] The group investigated four bioengineering labs situated on the campus of a major urban university, and sought to characterize the problem-solving and learning practices specific to each laboratory and across them, collecting an extensive body of data that included interviews with researchers at different levels of expertise, observations of their interactions and doings, guided laboratory tours, and eavesdropping on their research meetings. In analyzing the rich data set, we were intrigued to find in interviews the presence of emotional expressions as well as frequent instances of anthropomorphism, metaphor, abundant indications of creative model based reasoning, and complex forms of social engagement at the level of identity formations in interdisciplinary settings. Our analysis led us to develop an account of how the researchers' particularity – their personhood for want of a more adequate term, or "the personal" – is implicated in all aspects of science practice (Osbeck et al., 2011; Osbeck & Nersessian, 2015, 2017). The book that was one outcome of this study illustrated these personal or psychological dimensions of science practice, and concluded

[3] The research was supported by the National Science Foundation ROLE and REESE programs of the Division of Research on Learning: REC0106733, DRL0411825, and DRL097394084 (Nersessian, PI; Newstetter, co-PI).

with the assertion that *value* commitments were a glaring omission from the analysis we were able to offer. We noted that although questions relating to values clearly overlap with issues of emotion, identity, perspective-taking, and other topics covered, the topic of values was too vast and dense to take up with requisite care within the constraints of that project. Yet the topic of values remained as a promise to return to – a nexus of relation of all other dimensions of personhood and therefore science.

During the same process of analyzing the facets of "the personal" dimension of science evident in engineering practice, questions arose concerning the implications for my own discipline, how the "scientist as person" framework may be a helpful framework for understanding the intricacies of the practice of psychological science. However, I have spent too many years as a faculty member in a department historically dedicated to the pursuit of psychology as a human science not to expect fulmination against the comparison of psychologists to engineers. Some readers will respond with the adage that psychology is a human science and bioengineering is a natural science, and therefore their values are incompatible, even incommensurable. Others will wonder what all the fuss is about, and simply affirm that science is science, that science implicates an authoritative set of values, values that are therefore shared across contexts of practice, such as a search for truth and accuracy, systematicity, and rigor. In answer to both of these anticipated responses, one must note that there are various ways of understanding psychology's subject matter, as historical analysis certainly makes clear, and there are different models and conceptions of science and differing views of the relation of science to values. These questions resurface in the chapter to follow, but here it bears stressing that the divergent understandings of both the subject matter of psychology and the nature of science compromise straightforward claims about the scientific standing of psychology, and thus at a certain point the question of psychology's scientific standing itself becomes a question of value. Conceptual difficulties attend any attempt to demarcate boundaries between systems of thought as relevant to psychology, even in relation to a frequently taken-for-granted distinction between natural and human science that justifies the project of identifying alternative standards for human science research. I am inclined to agree with Plotkin that "it is no easy thing to distinguish between the natural and social sciences, and to say that here one ends and the other begins" (2002, p. 11).[4] Beyond this point,

---

[4] Moreover, there are important differences between physical and life sciences and inter-disciplinary science from either of these in isolation. These differences are at best ignored

I am concerned that the emphasis on *difference* between natural and human science – especially bolstered by the view that interpretive practices, empathy, or concern for complexity are required for the subject matter of human science – implies that "subjective" or "personal" human processes are *not* a resource for natural science. My fear is that this demarcation encourages a view of natural science as mechanistic and impersonal, a view at once inaccurate and unhelpful. To be sure, there is a need to consider the special features of the subject matter investigated in any inquiry, and to adapt goals, tools, instruments, and analytic guidelines accordingly. Yet there always appear gray areas of overlap; disciplines and the distinctions between them always reflect human decisions and human purposes.

Because of the difficulty in clearly demarcating human and natural science, and because the primary assumption guiding this project is that values are basic to the structure of any inquiry, this project does not take up the question of the scientific standing of psychology. On my view, the more provocative question concerns the relation between the humanities[5] and arts and sciences at the level of activity. Although this question has been addressed by various authors in different time periods, it has come back into focus in several contexts as a means of addressing the nature of creative and transformative thought. For example, Barbara Stafford's masterful analysis of visual analogy explicates processes of knowledge transfer through visual imagery, including artistic works, illustrated with historical examples (Stafford, 2001). Isaacson's enthralling biography of Leonardo da Vinci locates the roots of his subject's creative genius in his immersion in both science and art, or rather, his habitation at the juncture of these domains. In my own case, I have long been fascinated by the respective psychological arts of brothers William and Henry James, and in what I see as an underlying similarity or resonance in the themes of their work at different life stages, despite their different projects and goals.

It seems to me naturally that an emphasis on researcher as instrument, the psychological scientist as acting person, must lead us to seek better understanding of the interconnections of arts and sciences. There are of course many ways to take up exploration of the interconnections of arts and sciences and to consider their implications for psychology. My point is

or at worst intentionally and improperly erased in the service of a hard human science/ natural science distinction.
[5] I make this distinction with some trepidation, for there are of course many differences to be found in different branches of the humanities, and arguably between arts and humanities.

not to suggest that the domains are identical or equivalent, for there are obviously different goals and "degrees of freedom" attached to the activities in question (Bronowski, 1961/1956). However, in exploring interconnections at the level of activity, we might better understand the grounds for the generation of resources across domains, wherein may be found the possibility of collaborative, broad-scale interdisciplinary problem-solving and more complex and adequate models.

A note on the terminology to be used throughout the chapters is an important conclusion to this one. In the project of reenvisioning psychology's epistemic priorities and conceptualizing these as a set of activities, I use terms such as *person, observation,* and *sense-making* that have long histories in and beyond the discipline of psychology, and thus carry with them a great deal of conceptual baggage. *Person* and *observation* have been particular targets in historical and critical studies (e.g., Danziger, 1997, 2013; Longino, 1983), thus their reintroduction in the context of a discussion on values may strike one as unusual, even jarring. Discussion of persons, what we might call "person-talk," at least in in theoretical psychology, typically includes reference to one or more of the following: intentionality, rationality, language use, rule-following, or individuality/particularity, depending on the context in and purpose for which "person" is invoked. There are deep controversies across contexts: the meaning of rationality; the centrality of unconscious processes; the primacy of linguistic or pictorial expression; whether personhood extends to all or merely a subset of human beings, and on what grounds; whether personhood extends to conscious nonhuman beings; how "person" relates to "self"; whether just plain folks engaged in everyday activities or exceptional persons accomplishing extraordinary feats of creative achievement are prototypical persons; and how persons relate to the goals and methods of natural science.

But the major terms central to this discussion have multiple contexts of use and thus a variety of meanings. My intent is to explore meanings that have been less frequently emphasized, especially by psychologists, but that carry important implications. Thus, for example, with reference to "persons" and "personhood," conceptual and ethical difficulties abound, given the variety of contexts of use of these terms and the historical association of "person" with various forms of societal privilege (e.g., see Stam, 1998; Danziger, 1997, 2013). Yet, agency, intentionality, language use, and a unique phenomenological point of view are conceptually linked historically with "persons," and on the basis of these features a substantial body of theoretical literature seeks to claim a more central place for persons in psychology (Harré, 1992; Lamiell, 2009; Smythe, 1998; Martin & Bickhard, 2013; Martin, Sugarman, & Hickenbottom, 2010; Martin, 2017). No term is without its baggage, and therefore one might (as I do) use the term *person* with appreciation for the points of criticism raised, but with the intent to capture the particularized configuration of capacities and experiential core, the irreducible matter of "style" as it inflects even the most productive thought, as well as to emphasize the primacy of value.

The next chapter, *Science, Values, and Persons*, discusses the interrelation between the three topics named, and provides a framing for the subsequent chapters and the book as a whole. Chapters 3 through 5 each take up a category of activity and examine it in more detail, with focus on observing, imaginative sense-making, and perspective-taking. These chapters emphasize various meanings and suggest new ways of thinking about the value of the activity to psychology, for which reason it is here asserted to be an epistemic priority. The concluding chapter reiterates the emphasis on an acting person framework and on the project of reimagining epistemic priorities in accordance with it.

2

Science, Values, and Persons

It remained for a long time thus a mere sketched fingerpost: the perpetrated act had, unmistakably, meant something – one couldn't make out at first exactly what; till at last, after several years of oblivion, its connections, its illustrative worth, came naturally into view. It fell in short into the wider perspective, the very largest fund of impressions and appearances, perhaps, that the particular observer's and designer's mind was to have felt itself for so long queerly weighted with.
(Henry James, 1934/1909, p. 186)

OVERVIEW

This chapter offers a framework for understanding how values are "in" psychological science, and asserts that explicit discussion of epistemic values is vital to psychology's long-term viability and impact. The arguments are organized in three sections, in accordance with three interwoven goals. The first section discusses the meaning and schemes of categorization of values and points to controversies surrounding the distinction of epistemic from non-epistemic values. The second section considers the centrality of values in relation to a pluralistic foundation for psychological knowledge, with methodological traditions construed as distinguishable value systems with particular sets of requirements, from which questions follow. The third section emphasizes the importance of open discussion of value priorities for psychology, and forwards the view that generation of resources for flexible problem-solving and interdisciplinary collaboration are epistemic priorities in the context of global human challenge. The broader aim is to consider what values might be good for psychological science in contemporary social contexts, and what this implies for psychology's epistemic priorities. The claim forwarded is that an interactive set of *activities* is in need of greater attention and cultivation, that the activities in question are valuable across methodological traditions and across disciplinary boundaries, and that it is in these activities that the potential for generative thinking and collaborative problem-solving is to be found.

SECTION 1: VALUES IN SCIENCE AND PSYCHOLOGY

Among the first things new psychology students are taught about their chosen discipline is that it aspires to robust scientific grounding. The commitment to science as the epistemic foundation for psychological knowledge is reinforced within scholarly and professional organizations. The commitment is evident in the name and identity statement of the *Association for Psychological Science* (https://www.psychologicalscience .org/about) and is reflected in the fact that the second of five "core values" listed in the American Psychological Association's (APA) strategic plan is "Knowledge and its application based upon methods of science" (www.apa .org/about/apa/strategicplan/). A scientific foundation is central to the mission, identity, and overall orientation of most of those who claim to be psychologists. It is indeed of central value.

Yet to call a commitment to scientific foundations a *value* is mildly provocative, even jarring, for we are inclined to consider science and values to be of vastly different kinds, to belong to different categories, like "oil and water," as Longino suggests (1983, p. 7). Science is supposed to have nothing to do with values; it is to be an authority independent of agenda or bias, immune to the ploys of persons or the specific intentions of any group, other than the overarching purpose of revealing nature's secrets in the transcendent pursuit of truth. To be scientifically minded is to value "value freedom." Whatever difficulties such a view presents in relation to science in the abstract, the ideal of value freedom is especially difficult to uphold in the context of psychology's human service aspirations. To the extent that it retains a status as principally an applied science, a science dedicated to understanding human processes and improving human life, it is difficult to imagine how aspiration to a value-free psychological science is even conceptually coherent, let alone possible in practice.

Thus at the onset of our discussion we must recognize a tension in psychology's identity, for in seeking a scientific foundation, we inherit the legacy of a value-free ideal in connection with the idea of science. The representation of science as value-free in principle (i.e., as seeking value-neutrality as a goal) can be seen to be almost coextensive with the rise of modern science, given the emphasis on neutrality in landmark statements of the potential for science to make possible human empowerment and progress (e.g., Bacon, 1937/1620; Comte, 1957/1849; Mach, 1976/1905). We should note, in qualification, that there are important historically contingent variations in the meaning of value freedom (Proctor, 1991), and conceptual differences between, for example, autonomy, neutrality, and impartiality (see Lacey, 1999). Yet it is also only fair to note that the ideal of value freedom or value neutrality is rooted in the concern that values can disrupt objectivity, can lead scientists to see what they want to see, and thus to use science to further a personal, social, or political agenda: "[t]he notion that scientific reasoning should be value-free is often based on the worry that allowing values to influence science will result in wishful thinking" (Elliott, 2017, p. 13).

For contemporary philosophy of science, the expectation of value freedom is largely a thing of the past. Douglas notes that the philosophy of science community even as it developed in the early twentieth century displayed by and large a complex understanding of the relation between science and values, even among logical positivists. Max Weber seems to have been the strongest advocate of the value-neutral ideal for social science, and in this context the hope for value freedom in social science, at least as a philosophical project, seems to have ended with his death (Douglas, 2009).

Nevertheless, in the self-representations of psychological science, remnants of the value-free ideal deliberately persist or inadvertently linger. Precision of measurement and stringent experimental control have long been thought to hold the key to scientific legitimacy and elimination of the corrupting influence of values, especially when values are equated with personal priorities and meanings. Early and well-known examples include the effort to avoid commission of the stimulus error (Titchener, 1912) and the charge to restrict psychological data to publicly verifiable behavior (Watson, 1913; Skinner, 1938), despite the vastly different goals and methods of structural and behavioral research. In contemporary context the search for value freedom may be recognized in the search for material grounding through identification of neural mechanisms. The value-free ideal remains at the foreground of therapeutic practice through the affirmation of evidence-based practice as a general guideline for intervention, despite powerful arguments that the therapeutic enterprise is fundamentally moral, what we might call values-based at its core (Miller, 2004; Tjeltveit, 1999). Anecdotally, a reviewer for the proposal for this text noted that it

would be difficult to convince psychology students that values have anything to do with science!

It is against the "value of value freedom," too, that we can best appreciate psychology's preoccupation with questions of adequate method and
procedure. There is a long, strong tradition connecting psychology to
science, and science to a limited set of legitimate methods, and these
methods to the meaning of "being a psychologist." In the following example, Cronbach acknowledges that interests, instruments, tests, and concepts undergo rapid alterations, yet the relative stability in the methods of
inquiry employed by psychologists is identified as the qualifying criterion
of the psychological scientist. If we look at the implication of this statement
starkly, the identity of a psychologist is tied to a set of methods rather than
to a subject matter:

> The job of science is to ask questions of Nature. A discipline is a method
> of asking questions and of testing answers to determine whether they are
> sound. Scientific psychology is still young, and there is rapid turnover in
> our interests, our experimental apparatus and our tests, and our theo-
> retical concepts. But our methods of inquiry have become increasingly
> stable, and it is these methods which qualify us as scientists rather than
> philosophers or artists. (Cronbach, 1957, p. 671)

The prioritization and sanctioning of particular methods as a defining
feature of psychology, and the appeal to a logical foundation that justifies
this prioritization certainly are not without their critics. There also is
a lengthy history of passionate objection to the idea that psychology can
or should be a science like any other, and that its methods (e.g., experimentation) and goals (causal explanation and prediction) are fundamentally the same as those of other sciences. The objection found preliminary
but enduring form in Dilthey's distinction between explanatory and
descriptive approaches to psychology, with the related claim that understanding (others) is a process that draws upon the cooperative participation of the mind as a whole, the implication being that understanding is
required for the study of human experience (Dilthey, 1977/1894) . The idea
that the methods appropriate to natural and human science are fundamentally distinct or "bifurcated," and thus that they require fundamentally
different methods accompanies a parallel methodological tradition in
psychology, within which a set of critical frameworks emerged to contest
the idea that psychology's subject matter can or should be approached
through traditional natural scientific inquiry (labeled "positivist"). Giorgi's
(1970) description of the project of a human science psychology

(distinguished from the natural scientific tradition characteristic of psychology in the main, e.g., Skinner, 1938) was among the first to offer a constructive alternative to methods disparagingly labeled "mainstream" by the dissenters, and his approach was later joined by a proliferating array of variations and alternatives, including social constructionism, poststructuralism, critical theory, and feminist theory, with methods that include grounded theory, discourse analysis, and narrative inquiry and other qualitative approaches (e.g., see Wertz et al., 2011). These approaches have important differences in originating assumption and analytic focus, but they are united by opposition to what they call "positivism" and what they position as the mainstream of psychological method.[1,2]

Scientific Continuity and Values

As is attested to by the emergence of critical and oppositional positions, to claim that psychological knowledge proceeds from scientific methods is to raise more questions than it settles. At a most basic level, there are differing models of the logical foundation of science, each of which might be called "the scientific method," but which must be kept distinguished for conceptual clarity and methodological integrity. There are competing models of scientific reasoning independent of any disciplinary domain: inductive, hypothetico-deductive, Bayesian, and abductive models (Haig, 2014). There are forms and directions of inference specific to each model, and the frequent conflation of forms of inference is among the "bad habits of modern psychologists" described in a recent paper by Grice and colleagues (Grice et al., 2017). Second, there are differing ideas about how these various logical models should be understood, that is, differing conceptions of what science means. These involve differing understandings of how scientific thinking generates theories and how theories relate to "the world," to any hidden or underlying reality. These questions, in turn, correspond to differing notions of how we should understand scientific progress. Third, scientific concepts have multiple senses and cloudy meanings: fact, laws, cause, observation, explanation, measurement, and certainly "evidence" itself are all murky and multifarious and are the subject of volume upon volume of philosophical work spanning centuries. The entire

---

[1] Note that there are varieties of positivism historically rendered with important differences between them, and these have had different impacts on psychology's empirical projects (e.g., see Greenwood, 2015).

[2] For discussion of problems concerning designation of a psychological "mainstream," see Tissaw & Osbeck, 2007.

field of philosophy of science is dedicated to examining these questions – what science consists in, how its products it should be understood in relation to "reality," and the meaning of concepts central to any model.

Historical studies of scientific practice only amplify conceptual confusions concerning the precise nature of science practice. It is clear that no uniform, unchanging method may be charted even within the history of a single science, even a science such as physics, especially if ancient, medieval, and non-western scientists are included in the historical narrative. "One of the embarrassing results of this [attention to the history of science] is that those episodes in the history of science that are commonly regarded as most characteristic of major advances....do not match what standard philosophical accounts of science say they should be like" (Chalmers, 2013, p. xxi). The core of "scientific method," if anything, is construed as a set of rules for the measurement and manipulation of variables and rules for their interpretation, yet historians of science have not mapped these rules onto consistent procedures – a point at the center of Feyerabend's critique (Feyerabend, 1975). Sociological and ethnographic studies of scientific communities provide a more recent vantage point that similarly offers challenges to the idea of a uniform scientific method. Numerous broad scale empirical studies of scientists engaged in actual contexts of practice provide insight into how science proceeds and offer test cases against which a priori claims about science and its normative structures might be evaluated (e.g., Latour & Woolgar, 1979; Leonelli, 2016; Wagenknecht, Nersessian, & Andersen, 2015). On the whole these studies suggest variability rather than consistency in the understanding and application of central scientific concepts across specific sciences and specialties. Studies of interdisciplinary science practice in particular suggest that different scientific specialties demonstrate differing conceptions of appropriate and adequate scientific method, between for example, experimental biologists and computational modelers, in differing relation to the material constraints of their practice (Osbeck & Nersessian, 2010, 2017).

Demonstration of substantial variability across contexts of practice has tempted many to draw the radical conclusion that there is no distinctive, consistent feature to scientific method other than broad goals of knowledge construction. From this recognition of discontinuity in science, it can be tempting to leap to the conclusion that there is no principled means of determining the adequacy of methods, or to put it more crudely, that "anything goes" (heaven knows), whether in somber resignation or ribald celebration. This conclusion has indeed been reached by scholars, most prominently and provocatively by Feyerabend (1975), who argued that philosophers construct a rationale retrospectively to give the appearance of a common logic and procedure across scientific contexts. An emphasis on discontinuity is also a position associated with the "strong program" of social epistemology (Bloor, 1984) and other social accounts of scientific knowledge production from the past several decades (Latour & Woolgar, 1979; Longino, 1983), and the emerging interdisciplinary field of science and technology studies (STS).

It is important to note, however, that an emphasis on the discontinuity of science is itself a position that bears the mark of its historical situation. That is, the conclusion is not self-evident or even simply attributable to disciplinary perspective (e.g., anthropology, sociology). Lauden (1984) traces the emphasis on the discontinuity of science to developments in the 1960s and 1970s, during a period of transformation when views on science emerged that were fundamentally different from those of preceding periods, and these alternative views gained prominence during a period of social upheaval. Prior to the 1960s, he notes, both philosophical views of science and sociological views were essentially complementary, and both exhibited an effort to find a means for accounting for the extraordinary *continuity* of science over time and across disciplines:

> [B]oth sociologists and philosophers of the era shared a basic premise and a common problem. The premise was that science is culturally unique and to be demarcated sharply from other intellectual pursuits such as philosophy, theology, and aesthetics. The central problem each sought to explain was the impressively high degree of agreement in science. (Lauden, 1984, p. 2)

Lauden further notes that philosophers *and* sociologists prior to the 1960s were impressed by the high degree of agreement in science in comparison with other disciplines (their own!), and that the degree of agreement, the essential continuity itself became seen as the defining feature of science. It is of course, on longer view, the perceived continuity of science that grounds the idea that there is a consistent scientific method (e.g., Chalmers, 2013). Important to note from Lauden's historical analysis is that both continuity and discontinuity can be and have been read into the long history of science. The assumption of emphasis on either scientific continuity or discontinuity (i.e., a coherent or incoherent, consistent or inconsistent scientific method) reflects assumptions about the nature of science and the nature of human beings who practice it. Fundamentally, these emphases reflect differences at the level of *values*.

Definitions and Kinds of Value in Science

The ubiquity and inescapability of values and their meaning for the practice and products of science is a central question in contemporary philosophy of science (e.g., Douglas, 2009; Elliott, 2017; Lauden, 1984; Lacey, 1999a; Machamer & Wolters, 2004). For some authors, relevant questions concerning values and science have long moved past the question of whether or not science can be value-free to an acknowledgment that values are an inevitable, even desirable, facet of science, given that science is an activity or practice of human beings, for whom values are inescapable (e.g., Longino, 2004). Although there remains considerable disagreement as to the nature of the relation between values and science (see, for example, Lacey, 1999b), the intellectual project within philosophy of science has shifted to one that involves developing typologies of values and understanding, especially through case analysis, how different kinds of values can contribute productively to science, under what circumstances, and how values in science inflict policy.

Because of their ubiquity, values are rarely defined elaborately, beyond the simple acknowledgment that values are manifest in, for example, "what is felt to be important" (Machamer & Wolters, 2004), and that they are "something that is desirable or worthy of pursuit" (Elliott, 2017 p. 11). But the ambiguity affords multiple ways of understanding implications for science. Important to note, however, is that definitions of value tend to convey both emotional content and cognitive appraisal: a feeling of something desired and an evaluation that it is important or worthy – a *priority*. Values thus implicate desire and goal. It is easy, upon scrutiny, to think of "value" as a vague placeholder, a word used to express an ungainly morass of sentiment and judgment when no more precise concept is available. Yet this vagueness does not distinguish it from that of other fundamental concepts to which we repeatedly refer. It bears stressing that many concepts invoked for the purpose of pointing at something fundamentally important to our experience or acquisition of knowledge are almost insufferably vague, yet they still may serve important conceptual purposes. "Intuition," for example, is a word associated with a diversity of meanings, some of which stand in direct contrast to one another. Yet, philosophically, intuition, whether sensory or rational, has been repeatedly invoked to provide an account of epistemic and ethical foundations (Osbeck & Held, 2014). In comparing values to intuition, I mean only to imply that any concepts invoked as fundamental to all psychic life and activity remain fuzzy and elusive when subjected to analysis, unless examined within the limits of a particular context of use.

The vagueness of "value" prompts the development of typologies of value kinds, and descriptions of functions of different value kinds. A contemporary project is to understand what different kinds of values are operant in and can contribute productively to science, to be "good" for science. This is related to the task of distinguishing acceptable from unacceptable scientific values (Lacey, 1999). Values concerned with matters of truth or falsity, adequacy or fit of data, and the logic of inferential strategies are "epistemic" values (sometimes "cognitive," e.g., Lauden, 1984). The most strident defenders of the thesis of scientific continuity must admit that epistemic values are necessary for scientific progress, and that in at least a technical sense, then, the idea of value-free science is untenable. Yet after such an admission things become trickier. The contrast class of epistemic values is non-epistemic values, sometimes classified as social values -- but a kind of grab bag of "everything else" (Lauden, 1984): moral values, political values, practical values, aesthetic values. These value kinds are important to distinguish, and they relate to different concerns, even if the concerns are overlapping (e.g., between moral and political categories). Moral values, for example, might lead to reflection on the consequences of procedural or reasoning errors or commitment to avoiding fabrication of data; political values might entail commitment to giving voice to the historically disadvantaged; practical values might guide the development of easily administered questionnaires; aesthetic values concern the appeal of simplicity or coherence in theoretical systems.

Philosophers have noted that the boundaries are fuzzy, not only the boundaries between the various "everything else" categories of values, but even between the social and epistemic. The different "cuts" in values, the different strategies for parsing them by kind reflect different purposes, as does the prioritizing of some kinds over other kinds, as inevitably, if implicitly, occurs. Douglas demonstrates that the distinctions – the different ways the pie is cut – correspond to historical developments, locating the distinction between epistemic and non-epistemic values to 1950s philosophical debate, for example. Values themselves reflect social traditions and communal understandings. As one example, "how one interprets a cognitive value such as simplicity may well be influenced by socially structured aesthetic values, values that help one interpret and recognize simplicity" (Douglas, 2009, p. 91). There are also conceptual problems to be noted in relation to various classification schemes. For example, the classification of epistemic values as "cognitive" values has been criticized because of the implication that all other forms of value are noncognitive (e.g., values that entail moral reasoning) (Longino, 1996; see also 2002). Values also influence the typologies used, the classification schemes employed to distinguish values, and determine even the means by which values are interpreted, including epistemic values. Lacey, for example, while acknowledging that only certain values or forms of values are acceptable for science (e.g., empirical adequacy), acknowledges that "values contribute to some extent to the *interpretation* of empirical adequacy that one brings to bear on one's hypotheses" (1999a, p. 221, emphasis mine). There are also challenges to the idea that there can be any general and principled distinction between epistemic and social values, or any means of filtering and ordering social values to avoid contamination (Knorr-Cetina, 2013; Longino, 1983; Machamer & Osbeck, 2004).

Epistemic and Social Values in Psychological Science.

In relation to psychology, critical-historical and philosophical analysis of experimentation (Hoffman, Myerberg, & Morawski, 2015; Morawski, 1988; Robinson, 2014; Teo, 2018), variable-based research agendas (Danziger, 1990; Koch, 1993), and the conceptual basis of research divisions (Danziger, 1997) reveal complex intermixtures of social and epistemic concerns. In relation to clinical practice, pragmatic considerations relating to fundamentally social concerns factored prominently in negotiations that led to adoption of the scientist–practitioner model in psychology (Baker & Benjamin, 2000) and have been central to development and revision of diagnostic systems (Zachar, 2014).

Even more broadly, values of different kinds or categories are apparent in psychology's attitude *toward* science, marked by reverence and alliance, reactive resistance, or cautious, moderate, and skeptical restraint. These values inflect the practice and projects of psychological science at every level, from the collection of data to the methods used, to the interpretation of findings, to comparison of results in conclusion to one another and in the long view, as well as in assessments of the reach and limits of psychological science. As a recent example, values revealed themselves both in the project of seeking to reproduce psychological findings on a broad scale and in the range of reactions to the relative failure of this effort. The range or response extended from panic (the "replication crisis"!) to denial of any great significance associated with these findings (Maxwell, Lau, & Howard, 2015; Stroebe & Strack, 2014). Such reactions are reverberations of earlier calls of "crisis" in relation to psychological science and what may be seen as an emphasis on its deep discontinuities (Elms, 1975).

Psychology's disciplinary history reveals conflicts at the level of epistemic values, evidenced in its various "systems" or frameworks that endorse the analysis of different forms of data and different methods appropriate to those data. *History and systems* is an antiquated term in psychological science, rarely used in contemporary circles, but there is a reason the term was used as it was; the study of systems aided generations of psychology students in understanding the values guiding different approaches to psychology and the methods that correspond to them. As one example, Titchener described a division within empirical psychology between its structural and functional aspects, between concern for the "plan of arrangement" in the mind's "mass of tangled processes" and concern with the "system of functions" that enables the mind to "do" things for us or equips us to "do" (1899, p. 290), leading to the distinction between structural and functional "psychologies" (Heidbreder, 1933). The emphasis on structure required a reductive stance and prioritization of controlled experimentation; the emphasis on function required a systems level analysis and different methods, though systems level methods were not at that time precisely described. Functional psychologists considered structural psychology to be operating from the wrong scientific perspective, exploiting the wrong science for analogy: "The mind has been regarded too exclusively on the analogy of the chemical compound which is to be resolved into its elements, and too little as an expression of life to be studied in its activities," noted Angell (1915, p. 12). By contrast, the functional "attitude" is one that "brings the psychologist cheek by jowl with the general biologist" (Angell 1907, p. 69). The functional stance with its different epistemic values traded precise description of structural elements for a looser, fuzzier focus on dynamic interaction, in the service of a broader view: "Psychologists have hitherto devoted the larger part of their energy to investigating the structure of the mind. Of late, however, there has been manifest a disposition to deal more fully with its functional and genetic phases. To determine how consciousness develops and how it operates is *felt* to be *quite as important* as the discovery of its constituent elements" (Angell, 1904, p. iii; emphasis mine).

The *feeling* of what is "quite as important" in relation to the goal of understanding consciousness is a matter of epistemic *value*. As an epistemic value, it shapes decisions about what are to be counted as psychological data, how data are to be collected and analyzed, what will be taken as implications of the analysis, and how other psychologists using different methods (structuralists) are viewed. The alignment with general biology underscores that functional psychology is also a matter of identity for the psychologists involved, and their concern is with questions of social utility as well as epistemic integrity, complicating the project of demarcating the values involved in the "system" as epistemic or non-epistemic (Osbeck & Nersessian, 2015).

Overlap between epistemic and social values is also evident in expressions of deep dissatisfaction with psychological science that stem not so much from recognition of variety and discontinuity in its aims, methods, findings, or conclusions, but from concern that science is not adequate to address the vicissitudes of human experience. More extreme forms of this concern depict science and technology as ultimately a force for human harm, alienating us from one another and from the world, eventuating human destruction through weaponry, exploiting nature and hastening environmental degradation. At the risk of overgeneralization, these concerns may be found at the core of what has been labeled romanticism, marked by a celebration of irrationalism, divergent thinking, and authentic modes of personal expression (Berlin & Hardy, 1999). In the twentieth century, similar concerns and surrounding sentiments relating to science find expression in existential philosophy, phenomenology, critical theory, and poststructuralism. In psychology these concerns take form through the emergence of humanistic and phenomenological psychology. Objections to the effect that science sustains or cements existing power relations, economic disparities, and social hierarchies, at the top of which is the wealthy, white, usually Western male, are also of long standing. A related challenge proceeds from the claim that psychological science, like any form of natural science, is hopelessly ensnared in political and economic dynamics that illegitimate a claim to epistemic authority (e.g., Gergen, 1985; Parker, 2015). These critiques are aimed at the scientific foundation of psychology, but they are reflective of both epistemic and moral values simultaneously. The union of moral and epistemic values is evident in concepts such as "epistemological violence" and the critique and social justice stance that have energized a growing portion of the psychological community (see Teo, 2015 for review).

Critiques of this kind that focus not so much on the empirical adequacy of psychological science but on its dehumanizing impact and participation in perpetuating unjust distribution of resources and social hierarchies, though distinct in kind from questions concerning scientific continuity and consensus, intersect with and are in dynamic relation with epistemic critique. It is easier to make a case for the influence of political and economic control of psychology's disciplinary agenda and methods if one holds science to be devoid of continuity at the level of its logical structures. On the other hand, we can identify a "common horrified reaction to the abandonment of the idea of a universal, ahistorical method or set of standards, which sees the move as a complete abandonment of rationality" (Chalmers, 1999, p. 6; see also Proctor & Capaldi, 2006). I return to the point that questions concerning the legitimacy of science as a foundation for psychological knowledge at base concern questions of value.

PART 2: FROM VALUES TO PLURALISM

There is a seemingly insuperable conflict instantiated in the view of science as an ultimate human authority rooted in sound epistemic foundations and thus the only legitimate basis for psychology, and the view of scientific psychology as a bogus enterprise; a sham, even immoral. Bluntly, these are incompatible views. Can and should these views coexist, and with what long-range impact on psychology? Calls for pluralism in psychology (Koch, 1993; Kirschner, 2006) explicitly advocate opening psychology to alternative forms of inquiry beyond "the scientific method(s)," and signs of this opening are evident in many ways, including a name change for the APA division dedicated to issues of method from "Measurement, Evaluation, and Statistics" to "Quantitative and Qualitative Methods" (http://www.apa.org/about/division/div5.aspx). *Qualitative Psychology* is an APA journal exclusively devoted to qualitative inquiry, and coverage of qualitative approaches and mixed-method design in graduate research training is commonplace. Yet the conceptual basis upon which both traditional and critical/qualitative/alternative psychologies might move beyond merely grimacing and tolerating one another – that is, the grounds of fruitful collaboration and synergistic innovation – remains unclear, in large part due to the deep divide at the level of values.

It is fair to say, however, that the value divide reflects at least in part a series of mischaracterizations and misunderstandings. For example, there would be tremendous societal consequences were the epistemic authority of science to be not merely questioned but abandoned outright on a broad scale, for which reason the study of the conditions of science denial is crucial to our very survival (Gorman & Gorman, 2017). Closer to home, frightening implications for the impact on psychological assessment and intervention, education, child development, intergroup relations, and any host of other applications follow in short order. There is then, for good reason, legitimate and defensible concern over the abandonment of scientific rigor as a standard for psychological knowledge claims (Proctor & Capaldi, 2006). Yet surely some of the fear evoked in response to the idea of dismantling the epistemic authority of science springs from neglect of the important distinction between the possibility of universally and eternally binding scientific methods ("firm, unchanging, and absolutely binding methods," Feyerabend, 1975, p. 24) and standards of any kind (see Chalmers, 1999; Osbeck, 2005). Similarly, there is a great deal of misunderstanding surrounding terms such as positivism, realism, monism, and the relation between these, and the confusion likely contributes to the polarization. There is also much misconception surrounding pluralism itself, a failure to understand that much contemporary thinking in philosophy of science emphasizes that any complex phenomenon requires multiple investigatory vantage points and views in order to do justice to the complexity claimed, both in the natural world and human practice (Dupré, 1993; Harding, 2015; Mitchell, 2002; Nersessian, 2008). Moreover, what is frequently missed in psychological discussions is that there are different kinds of arguments in favor of pluralism, and differing forms of pluralism (ontological, methodological, theoretical); and that a call for pluralism does not require a call to anarchy, anti-realism, or an abandonment of methodological standards. Instead, it requires especially careful articulation of standards in accordance with specific aims and in relation to a given level of analysis. Nevertheless, in practice, epistemic values can be upheld within groups (e.g., methodological traditions, theoretical orientations) at the expense of another group and its values, resulting in caricature and misconception. This is not a problem limited to psychological science, and it is an underappreciated source of constraint on collaborative potential (Osbeck & Nersessian, 2017).

Values as Vectors

There is great merit to what some regard as a kind of middle path, one that finds a reasonable balance in the idea that standards may be locally established (relevant to the aims of the science and research project) but remain binding. They are enforced within the system (e.g., the particular science sanctioned within a particular historical period) in which the knowledge-oriented practice is situated (e.g., see Longino, 2002). It is in such a model that we can most clearly appreciate the central role of values in relation to any science, including psychological science. An earlier and highly informative but frequently overlooked version of this position is expressed in Gestalt theorist Wolfgang Köhler's analysis of the role or place of values in a "world of facts" (1938). The text is rich with insights and is worth reclaiming as a resource for confronting the value challenges and ideological divides psychology faces in its contemporary social and disciplinary contexts. Published during an era of extraordinary European unrest, Köhler's discussion begins by contrasting the public attitude toward science in the pre–World War I period, during which all branches of learning but especially science were held in "highest esteem," and in which the value of science was "too self-evident to warrant any argument in its defense," with the public view of science following the war, when "signs of a critical attitude became visible in several quarters" (Köhler, 1938, p. 1). The mounting doubt about the value of science after the war's devastation centered on whether science can adequately address, even dialogue with, "the essential questions of mankind" (Köhler, 1938, p. 1). Köhler's project, which he claims he undertook against the better judgment of his editor, was to articulate how values permeate science in all forms and at all levels, yet also hold the key to understanding the possibility of scientific progress.

Importantly for our purposes, the theory of values Köher offers is one that foregrounds *activity* and *persons*. Science cannot be purged of values because values are intrinsic to all we do: "At the bottom of all human activities are 'values'" (Köhler, 1938, p. 35). Science consists in a set of activities, including all the invisible activities subsumed under the heading of "thinking" (see Dewey, 1910), and thus naturally including all activities relating to science. In my view there is no clearer statement of the nature of values, yet also none that better represents why values are so difficult to discuss with clarity and remain elusive as a focus of analysis.

Values for Köhler are closely tied to what he calls *requiredness*; they constitute the highest human priority across academic disciplines: "The problem of value, or more generally of requiredness, is gradually becoming the outstanding difficulty or the eminent task of human thought" (p. 36). Requiredness is intrinsic to "all facts without exception in which there is an 'ought' or an 'ought to be'" (1938, p. 55). Facts subject to the principle of requiredness include all aspects of scientific practice: "There is no scientific procedure without at least the requiredness of logic, the distinction between essential and unessential facts, and so forth. A science, therefore, which would seriously admit nothing but indifferent facts even in its own procedure could not fail to destroy itself" (1938, p. 35). Köhler admits that general murkiness surrounds questions of value and requiredness in science, though scientific work "is utterly imbued with it" (p. 36).

Köhler seeks to avoid the pitfalls of either subjectivist (locating values in the "self") or objectivist (locating values in enduring and consistent principles external to any persons), individualist or collectivist theories of value, by viewing requiredness as a feature of a context or problem situation but relative to the specific aims that structure it – a relational phenomenon as it were, but not a relation of an unbounded or arbitrary kind. That is, there are no requirements that transcend particular values (analogous to "aim" or "goal" on pragmatist accounts), and no values without requirements. Values are most clearly understood as directions, *vectors*, a term Köhler willingly borrows from physical science to convey the idea that values are in some sense originating, and cannot be further broken apart ("split") or reduced to anything more primitive (1938, p. 336). This does not mean that all features of a situation (sometimes he calls this the "phenomenal field") have direction or directedness: "A coin before me does not point toward something, an interest does … Interest as a vector is experienced as issuing from a definite part of the field. If it is 'my' interest, it issues from that particular item in the field which I call 'myself,' not from a pencil to the left, not from a sheet of paper to the right" (p. 73).

A vector or line of interest may be qualified in various ways with emotional coloring – revulsion, affection, approval, which establishes the relation of subject to objects: "All however have this in common, that by such vectors the self either accepts or rejects the corresponding objects" (p. 74). Among the conceptual challenges Köhler's account presents is his use of "object" in reference to not only physical objects (e.g., a coin) but also attitudes, tendencies, or other persons. He calls his theory a relational theory of values, and it is this, but it is more precisely an interactionist view, or a transactional model of values similar to the transactional model of emotion developed by Dewey and Bentley (1949). The transactional view of emotion similarly offers a systems level view of what is traditionally theorized as an individual level phenomenon (emotion). It portrays emotions as posing demands that are real but always relative to a situation and system. For Dewey and Bentley, because actors in a system are always dynamically related to others, emotional expressions function as signals, and in so doing pose various forms of demand to other actors (e.g., to approach, avoid, provide care, protect). Emotions are indications of intimate participation with a situation or lived context (e.g., see Emirbayer & Goldberg, 2005). The demands are dynamic and bidirectional, constituting ongoing transactions within the system. It is in just this sense that we may understand values within the systems that constitute science. Values create contexts of demand – situations of requiredness within any context of inquiry (forms of data, methods of analysis).

Köhler gives few concrete examples to illustrate his model, but we might borrow from his studies on insight for clarification, because they help to us to visualize the basic dynamics and principles of his account of values with a highly simplified and accessible case example. Over twenty years prior to the publication of his text on values, Köhler undertook a series of studies on intelligence in higher primates at the Anthropoid Station in the Canary Islands, described in *The Mentality of Apes* in English translation (1973/ 1925). His interest was in the conditions under which primates exhibit acts that he labeled "intelligent performances" (p. 2) by solving specific problems. This example, of course, concerns the problem-solving behavior of primates, not persons, but the primate in question is an actor in a situation, with what we might identify as a goal, and something desired (fruit), which is at least analogous to something valued or felt to be important – important in that situation and for the agent involved. Thus the parallels are worth drawing for the sake of apprehending the structure of the situation despite obvious and nonobvious differences between primates and persons.

The experiments varied in details, but the studies of most interest employed a problem situation in which a desirable fruit was positioned to be out of the animal's direct reach (e.g., at a distance outside of the cage, hanging from the roof). In some situations, a "roundabout" route was required; other situations required the strategic use of implements (e.g., a stick, a stool). For example, a banana was placed out of the reach of the chimpanzee Koko (constrained with a chain), but a stick was placed within reach. On Köhler's account: "After some useless attempts to grasp it with his hand, Koko suddenly seized the stick ... gazed at his objective, then again let fall the stick ... then he suddenly took the stick again, and drew the objective toward himself" (p. 33). Variations in the experiment enabled Koko to employ different objects (a plant stalk, a stolen shoe, his drinking bowl) to extend his reach and capability. Whatever implements were used, their use gave them "a certain functional or instrumental value in relation to the field of action under certain conditions" (p. 36).

There is, then, a nonarbitrary relation between the goal (to obtain the banana), the stick (the implement), and the acts of grabbing the stick and using it to drag the banana forward, a relation that Koko grasps by means of sudden insight on Köhler's account. There are other possible solutions to the problem, but the possibilities are limited. It is not accurate to say that "anything goes." Koko will not reach the banana by hitting the stick on the ground, by chewing on the stick, by dancing around the banana, or by lying on the ground in denial of its lure. These are choices available to Koko in principle, but they will not meet the requirements of the problem situation for which the goal is reaching the banana. And yet, the requirements have no meaning independent of the situation and its structure. They are hardly "objective" requirements in this sense.

I am purposefully using the simple problem-solving situation confronting Koko in the roundabout experiments to make the parameters clear. If we move up to the level of the researcher's goals, we might similarly analyze Köhler's own research project, his attempt to understand the nature of intelligent acts in primates and its relation to the methods he used to study these acts. Although in this case there is a greater range of possibilities for action, greater degrees of freedom, the possibilities are not unlimited. As Chalmers (1999) suggests, the idea that the aim or goal of research determines the suitability or "rightness" of a course of a procedure (a method of data collection and analysis) is central to what is understood as a pragmatic account or knowledge or inquiry (James, 2002/1907; Dewey, 1938). Controversial though it has always been, a pragmatic account is one consistent with much contemporary thinking on the perspectival nature of science (e.g., Giere, 2010). What I am suggesting here is that epistemic values ultimately structure problem situations and establish a limited set of procedures capable of instantiating those values.

Psychological Methods as Value Systems

In addition to clarifying the important sense in which values infiltrate all inquiry (i.e., inquiry in general), Köhler's account of values is also helpful for conceptualizing the specific way values impact methods and practices within psychological science, specifically. For example, we may understand different methodological traditions and frameworks as distinct value systems, each with its own conditions of requirements and dynamical relations specific to that system as well as to the goals of any research project that embraces its values. Because values are primary, they precede even the questions we pose that serve as the basis for inquiry. Viewing methods as value systems takes into account that historical practices, assumptions, and associated values are part of the system, thus using methods does not amount to neutral, indifferent use of tools. Although a view of methods as value systems leads to endorsement of pluralism, it leads not to a pluralism that advocates annihilation of epistemic standards but, rather, to a pluralism that recognizes that different configurations of requiredness are applicable to different systems with different values. Norms within systems are binding, but they do not necessarily extend beyond the system in question, and certainly do not extend to all systems (e.g., all traditions of method). Importantly, too, no one value or even category of value (epistemic, moral, pragmatic, aesthetic) is ever operative, thus there is no one to one correspondence between a given value and a given method. Nevertheless, it is important to conceptualize the in-principle relation between values and procedures in any context of inquiry.

The idea that different methodological traditions within psychology constitute value systems with distinguishable sets of "requiredness" is one that has been expressed with other terms by other authors, especially in discussions of the function and viability of qualitative methods in psychology or the social sciences more broadly (Giorgi, 1970; Lincoln & Guba, 1985; Morrow, 2005; Ponteretto, 2005). For example, a recent task force directed by the APA to make recommendations on standards for evaluating qualitative research emphasizes differences in values, as values interface with broader philosophical considerations:

> Depending on their philosophical assumption, methods might be conceptualized variously and distinct sets of procedures might be valued. For instance, whereas some approaches prioritize the demonstration of reliability across investigators, others prioritize the depth of engagement. . . . . This diversity can create difficulties in the design and review process, as authors and reviewers are faced with research based upon a complex set of considerations rather than upon adherence to a single established set of procedures. (Levitt, Motulsky, Wertz, Morrow, & Ponterotto, 2017, p. 4)

I believe that we can draw from Köhler's insights and integrate the idea of "requiredness" with the idea that "distinct sets of procedures might be valued." In so doing we can see different methodological traditions (philosophical assumptions) as value systems with distinct sets of requiredness, and we can see that the requiredness establishes procedural priorities. In the preceding example provided by the task force, "depth of engagement" might be framed as the underlying *value* of the inquiry rather than a specific procedural goal. The underlying value (depth of engagement) limits the set of possible or legitimate procedural strategies, and the specific strategies have value only as they relate to the underlying set of values. I will not attempt to map the representation of "depth" onto a specific set of procedures, and I single out this particular value (depth of engagement) only for sake of example. For any given value, some methods are more suitable, and some are less so. For example, one might make the case that a count of behaviors does not meet the requiredness that follows a specified value of "depth of engagement" between researcher and participants. Therefore, counting behaviors would not be an appropriate method and would not constitute a legitimate method given this value, though there is no reason in principle why it would not be consistent with another value. Moreover, justification would need to be made for using fMRI technologies, regardless of the extent to which their use is more generally expected in contemporary psychological science. The point is that values pose constraints in inquiry, and constraints in turn contribute to methodological legitimacy. Constraints of any kind, by definition, run directly counter to a charge of "anything goes."

The importance of specifying values and analyzing the requiredness that follows from them is important not only for qualitative methods, of course. Although quantitative methods remain dominant across psychology, occupying a position of privilege, there is no one consistent or self-evident set of values underlying their use. Moreover, psychological methods, understood as value systems, are not static entities; systems evolve continuously with the participation of new actors and the creation of new demands, in keeping with new problems, new ways of thinking about science, and with developments in methods used by other disciplines. Even for the branches of psychology that identify more strongly with the natural science tradition and its methods, norms and procedures evolve over time, in line with new considerations, new conceptual goals, and new technologies. Vast sophistication and variation in quantitative analysis is evident since Cronbach formally recognized two stable disciplinary methods (Cronbach, 1957). Bayesian analysis, multidimensional modeling, and "big data" analytics are transforming psychology's statistical methods, are creating new trajectories of inquiry, and as these intersect with the extraordinary, explosive advancements in neuroscience technology, the discipline is in some ways hardly recognizable from the mid-century version Cronbach described. It is an open question whether the underlying value structure of quantitative psychology has changed, and in what ways, especially in comparison to the single-organism behavior analysis once prototypical of robust psychological science (Skinner, 1938), and against which many critiques of psychological science, including humanistic and phenomenological alternatives (e.g., Giorgi, 1970), were originally positioned. This point is especially important for qualitative researchers and other critics of "mainstream psychology," who may at times resist drawing finer distinctions between quantitative research goals or values in order to more sharply emphasize the differences between qualitative and quantitative research. At all times and for all psychological researchers, it is important to understand the epistemic values structuring the inquiry and to evaluate methods used in accordance with these values – the requiredness of the research situation.

Problems and Questions

In suggesting that methods are best understood as value systems, I do not mean to suggest that it is a clear-cut and straightforward task to distinguish value systems and to choose between them, or that the idea of a pluralistic psychology enjoys little resistance. In fact, the idea that different standards might be upheld by different communities of psychologists in accordance with different value systems (methodological traditions) is inherently problematic for those for whom consistency, reliability, and accountability are unqualified epistemic priorities (values), who may fear that recognition of methods as different value systems means little more than that procedural rules bend with the remover to remove.

It is a profound understatement to state that questions of this kind have created tensions and contributed to misunderstandings for psychologists concerned about questions of method. The controversies are more than matters of philosophical disagreement and affect more than the tone of communication at psychology department faculty meetings. They influence disciplinary policy, including the review and evaluation of psychological research, and thus establish psychology's possibilities for impact in the broader world. Yet the grounds for establishing and distinguishing any method as legitimate and therefore endorsing the value system that structures it are not easily determined. Relatedly, there are few grounds for establishing whether pluralism implies a limited or unlimited number of methodological alternatives and how these determinations are to be made.

These questions in turn relate to an even broader problem that is at the heart of some of the controversies over the claim that knowledge is relative to systems. That is, what constitutes a system, and where are its boundaries such that a set of values creates conditions of requirements in one system that do not apply in the other? Systems are embedded in networks; there are systems within systems, always. Methodological traditions in psychology may give the appearance of easy categorization into different systems with procedures and evaluative frameworks, but there are always questions and notable examples of overlap. Additional questions concern whether comparisons can be made between value systems on any legitimate grounds, and for what purposes. Does the claim of differing value systems imply incommensurability, in the literal sense of having no common measure (Kuhn, 1962), and what are the real implications of this implication? There is a long debate and large literature on this topic (e.g., see essays in Guba, 1990a), and it is taken up again in Chapter 5, in relation to the topic of perspective-taking and its function in psychological science.

We must also confront the troubling reality that in practice, at least in psychology, values are not equivalently valued. Psychology as a field of inquiry in the main places a higher value on generalizability than it does on depth of insight, places greater value on variability at the collective level than it does on variability in relation to a single life, places greater value on robust concepts than on discerning fine-grained cultural dissimilarities. These values are manifest and implemented in any number of ways, including the allocation of resources for research at levels of the department, the positions that open in universities, and the external funders that support their activities. Starkly put, institutional practices privilege, prioritize, and reward some research goals and methods over others, evident in everything from graduate admissions to peer review to hiring practices. These contemporary biases are deeply rooted in historical conditions, to the point of intractability. As summarized by Morawski:

> In its first century, the 20th, modern experimental psychology triumphed as the academic guardian of mental life. The experiment promptly became the principal method of inquiry, and laboratory standards of objectivity influenced sets for non-experimental research practices. The psychological knowledge ensuing from this scientific undertaking to calibrate mental life has deeply informed policy and institutional management as well as individuals' self-understandings. Experimentation reigns in the psychology produced in universities and research institutions and garners much of government funding for psychology research; its status surpasses all other contenders for the production of scientific knowledge about the psyche. (Morawski, 2005, pp. 77–78)

We are back to where we began this chapter – by pointing to the "core" value of central place of scientific methods as the source of psychological knowledge, and frequent assumption that this method is universal and ahistorical based on an underlying and transcended logical foundation. That is, although lip service may be paid to the importance of pluralism, in practice institutional factors prioritize one set of methods over others. These practices understandably can breed reaction, resistance, and resentment for those who do not cleanly fall in line. As a result, psychologists in different methodological traditions may merely tolerate each other if they do not engage in active opposition. In either case, there is little work toward mutual understanding let alone even cooperative, synergistic epistemic aims. At stake are essentially conflicts at the level of epistemic value: the "flourishing of charges and countercharges about truth and knowledge" turn "on assumptions about underlying values that are never brought into the light" (Kitcher, 2003, p. xii).

Yet if values divide, they also function to facilitate democratic and communal aims. Philosophers of science who study epistemic values emphasize the need for open communication and negotiation. Differing value kinds (moral vs. epistemic, aesthetic vs. moral), or different values within a value category (e.g., different epistemic values) require ongoing "judicial soul searching" and deliberation:

> [S]cientists typically value accurate predictions, clear explanations, logical consistency, fruitful research projects, honesty, credit for their accomplishments, health, economic growth, environmental sustainability, and global security. Of course, not all scientists value each of these qualities to the same extent., so we will see that they often have to deliberate about which ones are most important to prioritize in particular circumstances." (Elliott, 2017, pp. 11–12)

Open discussion of epistemic values (in addition to social, moral, even aesthetic values) is also essential to the application of science through policy making practices (see Douglas, 2009). This work, however, is rarely free of discomfort or conflict for those involved in open discussion and negotiation.

The open discussion of values is a topic that overlaps with the vast literature on reflexivity in research, defined broadly as "any turning back upon oneself or enacting any form of self-regard," intentional or not so (Morawski, 2005, p. 79). There are differences in how reflexivity is understood, the level at which it is applicable (personal or communal), and the role it plays in relation to scientific practices (e.g., Flanagan, 1981), but the general idea conveyed is that psychology's projects are enhanced by philosophical reflection and transparency, in full recognition that humans never enter research contexts without assumptions and agendas, and that failure to own one's assumptions fosters disingenuous research. Important to emphasize, however, is that reflexivity is not an excuse to assert a position without argument, or to shut down conversation or attempts at mutual understanding and negotiation in relation to conflicting values.

To the extent that there is a value for psychology to contribute construc-
tively to broad human problem-solving, the overarching goal of our disciplinary efforts – the requiredness of the broader value system – is not to
begrudgingly tolerate others in parallel play, or to perpetuate unhelpful
lines of division in the name of incommensurability. It is to work together
to common ends, and in the good of humankind, and more broadly, the
planet we inhabit.

C. PSYCHOLOGICAL SCIENCE: REIMAGINING EPISTEMIC PRIORITIES

Thus far, this chapter has sketched the broad parameters of several ways in
which we might understand values to be "in" psychological science, intrinsic to its practices, despite a long history of perception and sentiment that
science should strive to purge itself of values. I suggested a model of how
values function in psychological science broadly adopted from the Gestalt
conception of values as vectors, with "vectors" indicating that values have
directionality within a system and a foundational or primary status that
resists further dissection or reduction. As vectors, values establish a set of
requirements or demands in any context of inquiry, creating possibilities
for action (method, procedure) and eliminating others. I then suggested
that various methods in psychology could be understood as value systems
with distinct sets of demands, a claim that is very different from one
depicting methodological mayhem or anarchy. However, I also noted
several things that complicate the project of pluralism so understood,
one in which different value systems present viable options for psychological inquiry. Problems include, first, the difficulty in drawing clean lines
between systems, especially because value systems change as they evolve
over time. Moreover, in practice, some values are always prioritized over
others, establishing hierarchies that diminish the potential for a genuine
pluralism from which one might freely choose methods as appropriate to
values and questions. Against these problems, recognition that values are
inescapable in psychological science is necessary but not sufficient. There is
also a need for ongoing and open discussion and negotiation of values.

Note that in suggesting the value of open dialog and increased effort
toward mutual understanding, I am promoting a value that is itself not
specific to any single value system within psychology but extends across the
broad and divergent community of psychologists as a whole. In short,
although it is important to recognize different value systems with their
own requirements, we can also evaluate the requirements pertaining to

psychology as a discipline with a broader view, as a larger system. Therefore, in this section, I move from description of how values function to more prescriptive claims for the discipline. Specifically, I suggest a set of epistemic priorities across the different value systems within psychology.

Values "Good for Science"

The idea that open discussion and deliberation of values is an important task for psychological science accords with descriptions some philosophers give of ways various values are good for science, whatever the science in question. Examples include integrity and honesty (Lauden, 1984); democratic exchange of views (Longino, 1983); diversity (Harding, 2015); and even passion (Polanyi, 1974/1958). Questions about epistemic values overlap with questions about what is the "end of science" – the aim toward which it is progressing, and who should be the arbiter of its progress toward this aim(s) (e.g., see Kitcher, 1993, 2001). These questions are revealing of inescapable overlap between moral and epistemic values in any science, including psychology. What is the conception of "the good" that provides the basis for evaluating the extent to which psychology is progressing toward "good science?" For many psychologists, the idea of a unified theory is implicitly upheld as the good, evident in the many expressions of dismay at the discipline's fragmentation (Goertzen, 2008; Henriques, 2003). Other conceptions of good psychological science emphasize practical outcomes in education, clinical intervention, organizational functioning, and other contexts, and the connection between a unified theory and the potential for practical outcomes is emphasized (Staats, 1991, 1999).

Equally important though less frequently emphasized is the criterion of generating questions. Here is one view from the context of theoretical physics, in which the authors are responding to Popper's demarcation criterion to distinguish science from pseudoscience, whereby a science should be able to offer theories that generate falsifiable hypotheses:

> At best the criterion of falsifiability articulates the methodological perceptions of epistemologists, such as Popper, who were responding to the scientific developments of the first three decades of the 20th century within physics. In today's scenario of scientific developments, one might instead argue as follows: "It is much more akin to the implicit perception the physicists have of their own science," that without an active frontier full of new theoretical scenarii, theory–experiment interfaces and new probing research questions on the horizon, a science

would not be distinguishable from non-science. (Pandit & Dosch, 2013, p. 298)

How insights are applied, and the moral implications of their application, are also considerations we might think relevant to a conception of "good" science. Given the enormous complexity and differing trajectory of this question, it is one I shall bracket here. Yet it is worth mentioning that Pandit and Dosch note that their concern with understanding and promoting frontier science is tied to the project of imagining the conditions of possibility of a sustainable future for humankind, in which context they mention climate change and the challenges associated with the new information society as among the immediate crises requiring new questions and new theory. What is most remarkable in this call for an active theoretical frontier in the context of physical science is that it suggests that scientific goals, the end to which scientific progress is evaluated, must reflect and adjust to changing demands.

As noted, it is important to understand any system as evolving and transforming continuously with the dynamics of its internal organization and in relation to systems outside of itself or, rather, with larger systems within which it is embedded. Social systems, including disciplines, and including sciences, adjust to the entry of new actors and the departure of others, and transform with new configurations of demand. Thus our questions concerning the values that are "good for psychological science" should be phrased in a manner that considers our contemporary or present situation and context, as a discipline, within a culture, and with reference to the demands of humankind. To be consistent with the call to generate new questions and new theories in the face of new demands, we require reflection on the extent to which psychology's disciplinary emphasis on mastery of rules for collecting and analyzing psychological data functions to limit the range of questions that can be asked and answered, and whether these limits truncate the impact and viability of the discipline going forward.

There are notable examples of scholars in other disciplines reevaluating epistemic priorities in light of contemporary social challenges, as well as new questions that arise even in relation to standard methods and practices. Anthropologists Rabinow and Stavrianakis (2013) identify a need to better understand the analytic processes of their discipline, especially the basis of inferences made in the phases that follow data collection, practices in an investigative project undertaken in collaboration with bioscientists. They align their effort with Max Weber's charge for science to "meet the demands of the day," which concludes Weber's essay on the place and value of science in contemporary society and on the value of science in the scientist's life: "We shall set to work and meet the 'demands of the day,' in human relations as well as in our vocation. This, however, is plain and simple, if each finds and obeys the daemon who holds the fibers of his life" (Weber, 1946, p. 156). It follows an admonishment of those who seek to progress through "yearning and tarrying alone," and points instead to a need to "act differently" (p. 156). How to act is not a project Weber takes up with specifics, and neither does he clarify the demands one should rise to meet, leaving scientists to evaluate what is needed. For Rabinow and Stavrianakis, "the phrase meant that the process of bringing a complex experiment and experience to a close required more reflection as to exactly how to do that" (p. viii), in other words, "systematic efforts to think through our exit from 'the field'" (p. 7).

Rabinow and Stavrianakis do not explicitly frame their project in terms of values, but such concern is implicit, especially given its framing as a successor to an earlier effort to articulate the conditions of fruitful collaboration between human sciences and bioscientists, with an over-arching goal of designing practices that would contribute to mutual flourishing of these domains of inquiry (Rabinow & Bennett, 2012). The authors reveal their sensitivity to the interrelation of moral, social, and epistemic meanings by posing their orienting question as: "How is it that one does or does not flourish as a researcher, as a citizen, and as a human being?" (Rabinow & Stavrianakis, 2013, p. 5). Rabinow and Stavrianakis's reflections on what is required of them as anthropologists given the demands of the day (demands specific to their method and in the larger project of knowledge construction) prompt the question of how a discipline or any research project within it might rise to meet the demands of the day, and require reflection on what these demands might be "in human relations as well as our vocation" (Weber, 1946, p. 156).

A recent paper in engineering science is even more explicit in calling for a reevaluation of what is required epistemically given contemporary social conditions, relating these requirements to changes that have been wrought by human activity:

> Human activity, driven by science and technology, has built a new artificial world, damaging the planet's ecosystem significantly in the process. Systemic changes resulting from this activity, such as global climate change and poverty, are now central concerns while designing future policies and technologies that promote sustainability. The need to

> shift to sustainability-oriented design has led to significant introspection
> within the engineering community, with the recognition that engineer-
> ing practice needs to change ... This shift, in turn, requires
> a broadening of the engineering identity, and the way twenty-first
> century engineers are trained. (Date & Chandrasekharan, 2017, p. 1)

I do not think it hyperbole to suggest that the conditions in which we find
ourselves are unprecedented and overwhelming. We can name any number of recent threats to human flourishing as points of evidence, conditions
I noted briefly in the previous chapter: rapid and accelerating climate
change, global and domestic terrorism, information warfare unbalancing
political autonomy and democratic process, the threat of nuclear proliferation, natural disasters of outlandish and devastating proportion, contamination in water and food supplies, crippling poverty, apathy. As Pandit
and Dosch recognize, these are problems that threaten the possibility of
a sustainable human future: they present overwhelming, uncompromising
demands for every science, if not every discipline. The problems named,
individually and in combination, are numbingly complex; any lasting
solution will require multidisciplinary collaboration and cooperation in
the service of new solutions, even revolutionary forms of thought. There
are clear psychological dimensions to every problem named, and it is an
epistemic and moral priority to lend our instruments and resources to the
development of strategies for combatting them. What is even more intrinsically challenging than any of the problems named is that the age in which
we find ourselves, the day at hand, is one marked by uncertainty and
uncharitable transformation. We do not know what further challenges lie
ahead, and there will be devastations we cannot imagine.

The greatest resource in the face of uncertainty is active thought itself,
thought that is sufficiently nuanced to address the immense complexity,
sufficiently flexible to adapt to unpredictable and at times catastrophic
events, and sufficiently generative of transformative possibilities for human
life and interaction. In my view this requires a shift in emphasis, a shift in
what we envision as a priority for psychological science and scientists,
a shift to understanding the conditions that facilitate flexible problem-
solving, increasingly sophisticated modeling that adequately incorporates
personal and cultural levels of analysis, and robust, innovative directions of
interdisciplinary collaboration to represent multiple points of view and
develop new hybrid concepts (see, for example, Nersessian, 2008).
I suggest, too, that greater collaborative efforts within discipline, across
boundaries imposed by methods and value systems, are required for an

impactful psychological science. That there is of course an ongoing need for moral reflection in accord with new developments in thought and technology, especially in the context of discussions concerning the possibility of a sustainable future for humankind, is indelibly clear, but it is tied to the project of shifting priorities.

Activities and Persons

I end this chapter and begin the next section of the book with the question of what kind of activity creates the conditions that foster strategic interdisciplinary research, flexible problem-solving, the building of interfaces between disciplines, and the methodological interfaces within disciplines. A focus on *activities of persons* downplays the suggestion that training in procedural technicalities alone produces what is required. Activities of persons are broader than any method; they are more fundamentally expressive of our relation to the world and to each other. By better understanding activities – as enduring and holistic propensities – the possibility of transformative problem-solving is grounded. Activities are not matters of training so much as cultivation. This places them in the category of values – values to be cultivated in and by a scientific community, instantiated in education and what is emphasized and rewarded and encouraged across the discipline.

In the chapters that follow, I will explore three categories of activity that have broader implications for flexible problem-solving and transformative thinking: observation, imaginative sense-making, and perspective-taking, the latter being especially important for interdisciplinary science. I assume that the three kinds of activities are interactive, and that each fully integrates multiple dimensions of personhood: cognitive, emotional, social, cultural, perceptual. I do not in any way assume that these activities form a complete set; I set out only to provide examples in the interests of exploration.

Admittedly, there is nothing new or controversial in the claim that the activities named are the building blocks of scientific reasoning. However, multiple senses and uses are associated with each of them. By using the terms unreflectively, we can ignore important principles that I believe are crucial to a comprehensive understanding of science, and therefore to the long term strength and relevancy of any psychological science. Importantly, however, and perhaps most provocatively, as holistic human activities they may be seen to encompass both sciences and the humanities, or science and the "arts" writ large or small, despite the different goals and outcomes of scientific and artistic domains. They may be analyzed in such a way as makes their importance across disciplinary boundaries clear, which I seek to do. Thus we can draw from and relate the broader meanings to the goals of flexible problem-solving, multiperspectival and integrative modeling, and fruitful interdisciplinary collaboration envisioned here as disciplinary priorities. The activities in question follow from the act of establishing the acting person as the inescapable reality of science. That activity inevitably implicates actors, and actors implicate values, reflects a conclusion William James admitted to be "forced" on him "at every turn":

> the knower is an actor, and coefficient of truth on the one side, whilst on the other he registers the truth which he helps to create. Mental interests, hypotheses, postulates, so far as they are a basis for human action – action which to a great extent transforms the world – help to make the truth which they declare. In other words, there belongs to mind, from its birth upward, a spontaneity, a vote. It is in the game, and not a mere looker on; and its judgments of the *should be*, its ideals, cannot be peeled off from the body of the *cogitandum* as if they were excrescences. (1878, p. 18)

3

Observing

All of which gave me a high firm logic to observe; supplied the force for which the straightener of almost any tangle is grateful while he labors, the sense of pulling at threads intrinsically worth it – strong enough and fine enough and entire enough.
(Henry James, 1934/1909, p. 197)

'Actively believe in us and then you'll see!' – it wasn't more complicated than that, and yet was to become as thrilling as if conditioned on depth within depth. I saw therefore what I saw.
(Henry James, 2009/1909, p. liv)

The previous chapter laid the groundwork for the exploration of categories of activity fundamentally important across methodological traditions in psychology. This chapter takes up the first of these, emphasizing its enduring relevance despite controversies, varied meanings, and special problems related to psychology.

"Observation" is at the heart of classical or traditional understandings of science, tied to the conception of the empirical and the idea that knowledge arises through experience. Science proceeds on the back of evidence, and evidence is provided through observation, according to what Chalmers has called "a common sense view of science" (Chalmers, 2013, p. 3). Thus, observation presents some of the most important yet bewildering problems to philosophy of science, giving rise to questions concerning the nature of our access to reality, the contribution of the senses to knowledge, the nature of "facts," the possibility of genuine neutrality, the meaning of objectivity, the relation of the knower to the known. Despite immense controversy surrounding the concept of observation in science and philosophy, and despite special or particular conceptual difficulties attending the idea of psychological observation, or observation in scientific psychology, I suggest that the *activity of observing* is fundamental across methodological traditions within psychology, and even that it provides a deep conceptual bridge linking the arts and sciences at the most basic level of generative personal activity. "Observation," however, is frequently treated as a noun, disrupting its connection to human activity and the values that inevitably accompany it. I will therefore use the term "observing" wherever possible to underscore the active and inherently evaluative nature of the subject matter under discussion.

OBSERVATION AND PSYCHOLOGY

The following passage is typical of the way references to observation appear in the context of discussion of psychological methods: "[B]eginning in the nineteenth century and continuing to the present, there has existed much tension and debate concerning how well the subjective lives of persons can be studied by *careful scientific observation and analysis*" (Price & Barrell, 2012, p. 9; emphasis mine). Much is taken for granted in the tradition reflected in this claim, including the nature of scientific observation and its status as something that, in combination with analysis, gives rise to knowledge of a certain kind. Whether subjective lives are the kind of thing that can be studied in such a way is questioned, but not the nature and value of scientific observation itself as an epistemic category, let alone "observing" as an activity in a more basic sense. Instead, "observed" is used as an adjective, implying a straightforward and unproblematic equating of observation with "fact." There are references in psychological literature to "observed scores" on standardized tests, "observed behaviors" providing the data for functional analysis, observed patterns of neural activation, and so on. The meaning of observation, it seems, is generally taken for granted, though questions concerning the nature of psychological observation touch on the basic question of what should count as psychological data and what is the legitimate subject matter of psychology. In both classical/traditional (e.g., Thorndike & Hagen, 1969) and critical perspectives on psychological method (e.g., Gergen, 1973), we find discussion of "systematic observation" (usually of behavior), but the emphasis in the context of discussions of methods is usually on the systematic aspect, understood in terms of careful rules for procedure, and either lauded for its role in establishing control or critiqued for reductive implications alleged to follow (Osbeck, 2005). But the meaning of "observation" is murky at best, and at worst suggestive of naïve claims to a privileged epistemic access, or sensory experience devoid of meaning and interpretive stance (e.g., see Longino, 1990). Many, many critiques of this assumption of privileged access have been levied, against which the idea of observation seems obsolete and passé. However, just as problems arise from taking the meaning of observation for granted as the basis for psychological science, problems also arise from dismissing its relevance to psychology with charges of reductionism or naïveté. In both cases we overlook the embodied, goal-directed, value-laden, deeply human nature of observational acts, of observing as a habit and way of being, a vital contributor to the emergence of new ideas or the embellishment and refinement of existing ones. The problems of observation, of observing, are worth continual reevaluation and analysis.

The "Observer" and Early Experimental Psychology

The nature and limits of observation in relation to the psychological realm are central to the controversy surrounding the possibility of a psychological science, the project of an autonomous domain of study focused on experience. Among the most basic of problems associated with the concept of observation for psychology is the idea that knowledge arises through the sensory organs – through sense experience or sense perception, for which reason Bacon calls sense perception "God's lamp" (Bacon, *Sylva Sylvarum*, Century X, 900). Although on one hand the term *observation* is associated with the visual system (what is seen), on another view it refers more broadly to any sensory modality. In either case, if science entails observation and observation implicates sense perception, special difficulties are created for empirical investigation of mental phenomena. As an early critic put it, "in many contemporary lines of psychological investigation the so-called 'observer' does no observing" (Dashiell, 1929, quoted in Danziger, 1990, p. 97). An afterimage is "seen" in a different way than the object that induces it, if the image can be said to be seen at all. Reflected in the questions that troubled early psychologists is a lengthy and intricate philosophical history on the nature of perception and its connection to knowledge; the discussion took on complicated new dimensions as the possibility of a science of consciousness and mental life became more salient.

Wundt and his contemporaries also wrestled with the meaning of observation for the phenomenon of consciousness. Wundt scholar

Araujo's historical analysis reveals the complexity of the question of
observation as it related to early experimentation in psychology. Wundt,
reflecting assumptions concerning the nature of science widely upheld
during his time, considered observation proper to refer to the study of
phenomena present for the observer – things that are directly experienced
and not mediated by memory (e.g., Mach, 1976/1905). "Observation" was
reserved at the time for intellective acts by which the object of study
remains present to the observer – present in order that the phenomenon
under investigation may be studied for its properties and compared with
other things. Thus on Araujo's account, Wundt wrestled with the idea that
genuine self-observation might be "an illusion" (Araujo, 2016, p. 177),
noting Wundt's admission that "the psychologist who wants to fix his
consciousness will eventually perceive only this one curious fact: that he
wants to observe"[1] (Wundt, 1882, p. 395, cited in Araujo, 2016, p. 177;
emphasis mine). If a phenomenon is ephemeral, we require memory to
reproduce it, wherein lies opportunity for distortion and inaccuracy.[2]
The extensive, repetitive training required of early psychologists – training
to become even adequate experimental subjects – can be best understood
against the goal of making progress toward genuine self-observation, to try
to minimize distortion to the extent possible.

As is well known, the training and ongoing work of early experimenters
included the continuous interchange of roles or positions, a series of
rotations between experimental tasks peculiar to the study of consciousness. Danziger thus characterizes the "observer" term as a social identity
within the experimental situation of early psychology laboratories and
a "strictly intraexperimental identity," connected to playing a particular
role in the situation of the experiment. Yet the use of the term *observer*, like
subject, was not used in a consistent or facile manner:

> In the first place, the history of experimental psychology is marked by
> a long period of indecision about the appropriate way to refer to the
> experimental identity of those who functioned as the source of data.
> In the very early days of the discipline a number of terms were in use, . . .
> but in the English-language literature two terms quickly overshadowed
> all the others: "subject" and "observer." By the end of the nineteenth

[1] As Araujo acknowledges, both Kant and Comte were dismissive of the possibility of
inner observation, referring to the idea that the act of observing consciousness "interferes
and modifies that which should be observed, thus invalidating the procedure" (Araujo,
2016, p. 176f).
[2] The problem of temporality confronting the idea of observing conscious phenomena was
a problem also obvious to William James (2007/1890).

century the former was being used in about half of all published reports, and the latter in about a quarter. But then it took another half-century for the use of observer to dwindle to a negligible level. Clearly the connotations of these terms were not a matter of indifference at the time but presented authors and editors with a real choice.

(Danziger, 1990, p. 95)

In Danziger's view, the "ideological connotations" of *observer* (like those of *subject*) were "probably salient only for a minority of experimentalists" (1990, p. 97). He acknowledges, however, that the use of the term was problematic and tied to the eventual reaction of behaviorists, contributing to controversy and eventual divides within the discipline. Watson (1913) took direct aim at the idea that mental states could be observed, and at the ancillary assumption that failure to replicate or reproduce findings is a problem rooted in the training and skill of the observer, by which observers must be trained to observe. By contrast, Watson argued, physics and chemistry first look for shortcomings in the experimental setup – the situation – rather than in the training of the researcher:

Psychology, as it is generally thought of, has something esoteric in its methods. If you fail to reproduce my findings, it is not due to some fault in your apparatus or in the control of your stimulus, but it is due to the fact that your introspection is untrained. The attack is made upon the observer and not upon the experimental setting. In physics and in chemistry the attack is made upon the experimental conditions. The apparatus was not sensitive enough, impure chemicals were used, etc. In these sciences a better technique will give reproducible results. (Watson, 1913, p. 163)

In view of what he regards as a fundamental difference between psychology and physical science, Watson's solution is to alter psychology at the level of both object and method of study in order to attain the goal of genuine observation, by which it must abandon the idea of mental states as scientific objects: "The time seems to have come when psychology must discard all reference to consciousness; when it need no longer delude itself into thinking that it is making mental states the object of observation" (Watson, 1913, p. 163). The well-known strategy to restrict psychological data to observable behavior, with "observable" meaning publicly verifiable, open to disconfirmation, on the one hand restored "observation's" direct tie to the sensory organs: behavior could be plainly "seen." Yet what was to be counted as "seeing" was the collective process, collective sense experience we might say, in line with the conception of science to which Watson aspired (Comte, 1957/1849; Mach, 1976/1905).

For psychology, a fallout of the shift in emphasis from consciousness to behavior as the focus of psychological inquiry is that the personal contribution of the psychological researcher to the experimental situation – the acting person – is effectively removed. In Danziger's analysis, the term *observer* was the topic of ideological debates among experimental psychologists in the 1920s, centered on the extent to which the term *observer* remained meaningful in relation to all developing trajectories of psychological research. At least one voice in the conversation derided the "cult of objectivism" that would eliminate "observer" from the lexicon, failing to recognize the importance of experiments by which "the organism enters the scene as an *agent*" (Bentley, 1929, quoted in Danziger, 1990, p. 97; emphasis in the original).

The idea that replicability and rigor are rooted in the experimental setup rather than in the cognitive processes of the observer is not limited to the experimental analysis of behavior. In correlational research, an analogous emphasis is to be found in the focus on the features of measurement instruments – the psychometric properties of tests and standardized procedures for administration. In both experimental and correlational research, the emphasis is on the application of rules – rules for defining, measuring, manipulating, and interpreting. Among the "epistemopathic peregrinations of the inquiring impulse," Sigmund Koch derided psychology's "tendency to accept on authority or invent a sacred, inviolably 'self-corrective' epistemology that renders all inquiry in the field a matter of application of rules which preguarantee success," along with "a view of all aspects of the cognitive enterprise as so thoroughly rule-regulated as to make the role of the cognizer superfluous" (Koch, 1981, p. 258). There is an important sense in which the loss of the "cognizer" is a loss of the "observer" – the researcher and theorist who retains other identities and approaches any research task with feelings, relationships, shared agendas, and personal goals – a subjective presence. As others have noted in different ways, a focus on instrumentation and method directs attention from the ultimately creative and agentive acts in which evidence is defined, amassed, and used to various ends.

Thus at a most fundamental level, to appreciate the role of the acting person in psychological science requires a fresh look at observation, or more accurately, at the activity of observing.

PHILOSOPHICAL CONCEPTIONS OF OBSERVATION:
PROBLEMS AND PROMISING DIRECTIONS

Before proceeding, it is important to acknowledge several broader philosophical problems that relate to observation in general, problems that are not confined to the special problem of observation of psychological phenomena. There are stubborn glitches relating to the conception of observation, its relation to experimentation and theory that both precede and exceed the problem of psychological observation specifically. I will distinguish these as (1) the questionable importance of sensory contact to "observation," (2) the tangle of observation and theory, and (3) the questionable reliability of "naked-eye" observation, a topic closely related to (1) and (2).

(1) The Questionable Importance of Sensory Contact to "Observation"

Among the most basic of difficulties is the relation of observation to sense perception. The issue at stake is essentially as follows: if observation provides the evidence upon which theory is grounded, science is built upon the shakiest of grounds. Observation repeatedly has been demonstrated as a questionable and unreliable epistemic guide. Moreover, the role of the sensory organs in science, direct sensory contact with the object of interest, is of limited use in sciences such as theoretical physics. Almost invariably, science involves the use of instruments designed for the purpose of tracking and measuring; these alter the position and relation of the observer to the observed, modifying the nature of the sensory contact, whether the instrument in question is a telescope or questionnaire. Theoretical progress, indeed, is often gained by abandoning reliance on the senses, beginning at least with Copernicus, who was to "exchange his actual terrestrial station for an imaginary solar standpoint" – removed, that is, from the sensory information provided through his situation on earth, by means of which the sun appears to cross the sky (Polanyi, 1974/1958, p. 2). Contemporary physicists reference observation in relation to detection of information not visible to the naked eye – using receptors that record electromagnetic interactions and by extension reveal the presence of interacting entities. But the entities themselves are infrequently known through direct sensory contact. Shapere's (1982) classic paper on the concept of observation in philosophy thus distinguishes the "philosopher's observation" (an observer makes contact with phenomena by means of direct sensory perception) from astrophysicists' observation (an observer

makes no direct sensory contact with phenomena but detects patterns of
interaction through highly specialized equipment). Hacking, similarly,
acknowledges that observation through sense perception plays
a relatively limited role in scientific practice, or at least a minor role in
experimentation. "Some great experimenters have been poor observers,"
he notes, and "often the experimental task, and the task of ingenuity or
even greatness, is less to observe and report than to get some bit of
equipment to exhibit phenomena in a reliable way" (Hacking, 1983,
p. 167). Haig (2014) provides a helpful discussion of the meaning and role
of detection in psychological science, noting the importance of distinguishing between detection and explanation, and the value of detection and of
robust generalization in its own right, apart from theories of cause (explanatory): "The successful detection of a phenomenon is an important
achievement in its own right, and a significant indicator of empirical
progress in science" (p. 57). Haig notes that psychologists in particular
have insufficiently accounted for the role of detection in empirical progress, prompting not only a too heavy-handed emphasis on explanations
(search for mechanisms) but also a critical response that fails to distinguish
the two activities.

(2) The Tangle of Observation and Theory

A second and related controversy concerns the relation between observation and theory, specifically around the presumption that observation can
be conducted neutrally, without commitment to value, agenda, desire, or
theory. These are not new concerns by any means, being that they were
raised in analogous form in the nineteenth century in Whewell's depiction
of knowledge as a commixture of "thoughts and things" (1844) and, much
earlier, implied in Bacon's description of "idols of the theater" – forms of
bias that originate in doctrine and ideology (1937/1620). However, concerns
intensified in the twentieth century and in one form or another became
a prominent theme in much philosophy of science. The critique is linked to
arguments both logical and empirical, the former emphasizing the reliance
of observational reporting on the forms of language available to the
observer, which vary with context and culture; the latter consisting of
evidence provided by anthropological research and psychological studies
of visual illusion and by historical studies of science. Hanson's *Patterns of
Discovery* (1958), most readily associated with the idea that observation is
laden, loaded, or saturated with theory, begins not with an abstract treatise
on the nature of observation but with a study of the particular case of

particle theory. Through this case study Hanson articulates reasons why the traditional separation of observation from theory is untenable or incoherent across the sciences, given the "interplay between facts and the notations in which they are expressed" (1958, p. 2). Hanson's focus is the discovery process, what he calls *theory-finding*: "Let us examine not how observation, facts, and data are built up into general systems of philosophical explanation, but how these systems are built into our observations, and our appreciation of facts and data" (p. 3). The examples Hanson provides in his chapter on observation make clear that he regards the selection of relevant facts and the posing of questions in any observational instance to reflect the interests and starting assumptions of the observer – what we might call *values*. The relevant question, however, is not only how theoretical stance influences what is observed, but whether observers observe the same phenomenon, given that "seeing" is an experience, not itself the physical process of retinal reaction to a physical stimulus. Hanson's answer is complex, and his project is one of illustrating the complex intertwining of language systems, expectation, and essentially nonrational considerations with the coordinated acts of theory development.

The broader implication of Hanson's analysis may be simply that observation requires a theory that makes sense of it (Hacking, 1983), a position adopted freely in much of contemporary physics, namely, that "it is the theory which decides what can be observed" (Heisenberg [paraphrasing Einstein], quoted in Pandit & Dosch, 2013, p. 38). It is important to recognize, too, that "theory" is used loosely in defending the basic claims articulated by Hanson. It is certainly the case that one cannot remove ideas or assumptions from acts of observation, but it is another thing to suggest that all researchers hold a developed theory and implicitly seeks to confirm it through observation, or that developed theory is necessary to all acts involved in observation. Shapere, for example, provides the example of a lab assistant trained to count instances of an interactive phenomenon using specialized equipment designed for the purposes of detection. She may lack a developed theory of the reason for the interaction or even an understanding of the entities presumed to interact, yet her detection skills may be well honed, accurate, and reliable, in which case we would need to consider her an effective observer (Shapere, 1982). Volumes have been written in critique and defense of the meaning of theory-laden observation, and which relate this to the idea of social construction. A helpful middle ground may be found in Sabina Leonelli's philosophical analysis *Data-Centric Biology*, which points to the futility of searching for "mind-independent" data in biology – data independent of the meaningful purposes. She offers what she terms a *relational view* of data, and ties them not only to conditions of their original use but also to repackaging and repurposing, wherein data may be used again and again, passed between researchers, aligned with different goals. They are not free-floating bits of "evidence" that demonstrate their own relevance. They have no "fixed independent value" outside of particular problem-solving activity (Leonelli, 2016, p. 70). In a broad sense, there are obviously theories at play, or at least ideas about how what is detected will be useful.

(3) The Questionable Reliability of "Naked-Eye" Observation

In contemporary philosophy of science, observation has recently received greater attention as an epistemic category after a period of relative neglect, with work that includes both historical reflection and contemporary analysis of its important features. Experimentation is usually viewed as an extension of observation, as mediated or mediating observation rather than "direct" observation traditionally associated with immediate "sight," even sensory intuition (Osbeck & Held, 2014). Mediated observation contrasts with "naked-eye" observation, leading to what sometimes results in a downplaying of the active role of the former, a holdover from what was sometimes held as a distinction between observation as passive sensory recording – receiving impressions – and the active manipulation accomplished experiment (Hudson, 2014).

Reasons to consider naked-eye observation a dubious epistemic foundation are many, represented by, as one example, the fact that naked-eye observation led to the conclusion that the sun revolves around the earth. Nevertheless, it is "our first and most important observational method" that "forms the empirical basis for all our interactions with the world" (Hudson, 2014, p. 231). Naked-eye observation remains "a highly preserved and informative (albeit primeval) methodology . . . whose reliability no-one rejects" on a basic day-to-day level, as a basis for getting along and around in the world: "objects revealed by such preserved methods enjoy a prima facie claim to reality that counterweighs the negative historical induction that would lead us to assert their nonreality" (p. 235). Hudson notes as an example that "we continue to observe the thoroughgoing solidity of chairs and tables despite an atomic theory that tells us to regard such objects as mostly empty space" (p. 235).

Our everyday reliance on naked-eye observation may help to account for the allure of naked-eye observation in psychology's epistemic history:

naked-eye observation of behavior trumping "unobservable" introspective facts, and what *appears* to be naked-eye observation of brain states made possible through neuroimaging. Although the images are in fact complexly mediated by technology, data provided through neural activation technology remain compelling to psychologists because of the imagery available to the naked eye: there it is – we are "seeing" the brain! There is an emotional appeal to naked-eye observation, an "irrevocable attachment" (Hudson, 2014, p. 247) or at least affective pull, that perhaps exceeds its epistemic affordances.

REENVISIONING OBSERVATION: "BEING OBSERVANT"

Hacking notes that although naked-eye observation is less important to science than philosophers have tended to depict it, there is a form or sense of observation that is necessary for what we might conceive of as innovative science. He calls this "a more important and less noticed kind of observation that is essential to fine experimentation," noting that "the good experimenter is often the observant one who sees the instructive quirks or unexpected outcomes of this or that bit of equipment." It is, Hacking notes, this speed and ease of "seeing" the unexpected that underlies discovery: "Sometimes persistent attention to an oddity that would have been dismissed by a lesser experimenter is precisely what leads to new knowledge." This is observation, for Hacking, but not the classic sense of observation as sense-experience providing the basis for theory formation, through a passive recording of sensory data, an indiscriminate recording, a stamping in wax. The activity in question "is less a matter of the philosopher's observation as reporting what one sees," he notes, "than the sense of the word we use when we call one person observant while another is not" (Hacking, 1983, p. 167).

At its base naked-eye observation involves a noticing of similarity and difference, a basic comparative act and detection of pattern that can be perhaps infinitely extended with additional discriminations. Such attention to particular features of situations is, however, not an activity limited to discrimination of sound or color. There is a broader notion of observation or observing that is important to discern here, yet it is one rarely acknowledged openly as important to psychological method. Hacking acknowledges, too, that this is a sense of observation that is more in keeping with contemporary physics than it is with positivism. He connects the basic activity of noticing and distinguishing, unique to each person – each observer – with his interest in

Bacon's depiction of "prerogative instances": "striking and noteworthy observations," "fingerposts" that "afford very great light." The insights do not always hold up when subjected to test – fingerposts can mislead the observer, but they provide the grounds of possibility for important insight. According to Hacking's analysis, fingerposts are not so much given as sought, and are revealed only through directed effort. He relates this activity to Bacon's metaphor of the bee in Book One of *Novum Organum*. Bacon contrasts the bee with the ant and the spider in relation to different approaches to science, and sees progress only in relation to the bee.

> Those who have handled sciences have been either men of experiment or men of dogmas. The men of experiment are like the ant, they only collect and use; the reasoners resemble spiders, who make cobwebs out of their own substance. But the bee takes a middle course: it gathers its material from the flowers of the garden and of the field, but *transforms and digests it by a power of its own*.
>
> (Bacon, *The New Organon* [Book One], 1620; emphasis mine)

In the reference to transforming and digesting material "by a power of its own," there is a clear implication in Hacking's analysis of Bacon's metaphor that the agentive activity of observing is responsible for genuine progress in science, an emphasis that accords with Polanyi's depiction of the personal dimension of observational activity, for example in reference to "the *pouring out of ourselves into the particulars* given by experience so as to make sense of them for some purpose or in some other coherent context" (1974/1958, p. 61; emphasis mine).

Both Hacking and Polanyi imply that there is a skill to observing, that proficiency can be to some extent acquired, yet they also both note that some persons, naturally, are better at observing than are others. Similarly, William James described discrimination as an ability more naturally developed in some persons but amenable to improvement with intentional, directed effort (1890). Observation is rooted in the particularities of persons as much as in the particularities of situations observed. Some persons have cognitive faculties that incline them toward discrimination and noticing of differences. Precision of focus, moreover, requires facility of expression, the ability to communicate in words the different features of which the observer makes painstaking note. The language used must be adequate to the goal. All of this begs the question of the relation of observation to language, the role of rhetoric in science, and other cumbersome topics that have occupied the concerns of philosophers of science for much of the previous century, all of which, in turn, implicate the complex capacities of persons.

Moreover, what is picked out and noticed will vary with the interests, goals, native abilities, learning history, cultural and linguistic resources, emotional state, and social positioning of the observer: observation is rooted in the particularities of persons as much as in the particularities of situations observed. Yet Hacking also emphasizes that observation is enhanced and extended by knowledge; experience in a domain makes possible the noticing and discrimination of finer and finer difference and detail, consistent with the view that intuition of a certain kind increases with expertise (see Cokely & Feltz, 2014, for review). One may notice different features, different patterns at different times, corresponding with different physiological or emotional states, preoccupations, priorities. However, observation is unlikely to improve in conditions of fatigue, inattention, or neglect, thus the habits, states, skills, and proclivities of the observer assume a place of inestimable importance.

The idea of observation as an activity of informed and engaged "noticing" finds precedent in a broader history of observation and observation-related concepts. Despite variety in meanings, the fundamental importance of observation across scholarly domains is emphasized repeatedly in various ways. I review some of the important insights in the following section, not with the goal of establishing some concept of observation as a binding one, but in order to highlight aspects of observation that have been overlooked in prioritizing the experimental situation (or the specific procedures of any method) over the embodied cognitive agent (the scientist).

OBSERVATION AS "THE UNIVERSAL SPIRIT OF THE ARTS AND SCIENCES"

The place of observation in the history and philosophy of science, and the relation of observation to other epistemic practices such as experimentation, is highly complex, with confusion arising in some cases from mistranslation and in other cases from taking the meaning for granted in connection with the concept of evidence or facts, as earlier noted. In historian Gianna Pomata's analysis, many instances of what has been translated as "observation" (e.g., infamous passages in Bacon's *Novum Organum*) are actually *experimentum* or *experientia* (Pomata, 2011, p. 46). According to Katherine Park, the Greek word *tērēsis* that was translated into Latin as *observatio* appears only in Aristotle's *History of Animals*, and therein not as an epistemic category corresponding to the careful act of describing animal habits but, rather, in association with certain forms of animal behavior, most notably an attentive state of "keeping a watch," invoked for a description of a spider in relation to potential prey:

> *It always builds its web over hollow places*
> *inside of which it keeps a watch on the end-threads, until some creature*
> *gets into the web and begins to struggle, when out the spider pounces.*
> (Aristotle, *History of Animals*, Book IX, 39, in Ross, *Complete*
> *Works of Aristotle*, p. 1764)

Park suggests that "watching and attentive waiting" is the root or core of observation in this sense. This watching and attentive waiting is an active state rather than a passive occupation – there is prey at stake in the attentive watching, but it is a state of heightened focus, one on which the spider's existence may be seen to depend. *Observatio* and cognate terms were at the time used with reference to human activity only in relation to the study of the stars, in relation to the activity of watching (the heavens) and interpreting natural signs and connections between signs and events, such as the temporal relation of thunder and rain. These activities served predictive purposes relating to agriculture and navigation, activities that for the human are as necessary to survival as is the spider's vigil for its prey. Of interest, too, the Greek and Latin forms of *observatio* are also the root of "observance" – as of a ceremony, custom, or law (Park, 2011). Later translations of relevant passages in Aristotle's *Posterior Analytics* and Bacon's *Novum Organum* are, according to Pomata's analysis, mistranslations.

Over time, "observation" took on epistemic connotations and became what Pomata calls an "epistemic genre" in its own right, but this came about slowly. Sometime between the seventeenth and eighteenth centuries, "observation" was more widely adapted in contexts of natural philosophy, and this because, to quote Pomata, it was "newly interpolated into the standard Aristotelian vocabulary of experience, of which previously it had never been part" (Pomata, 2011, p. 66). This usage was widely adopted by followers of Aristotle, including William Harvey, who added "diligent observation" to the conditions for the acquisition of "true knowledge," noting that "in every discipline diligent observation [*diligens observatio*] is required" (quoted in Pomata, 2011, p. 80; footnote 119).

During the sixteenth century, references to *observationes* – the plural form, and a noun – appeared in titles of works across many fields, and persons began to *identify* as *observationes* (observers) (Pomata, 2011).

In medicine, the writing of self-identified observers began to be assigned to students to encourage them, to give them models, for describing the particularities of a given case, to write a clinical history, as it were. What Pomata considers a "turning point in the early history of the genre" (2011, p. 49) was Mario Niolio's sixteenth-century publication of the observations of astronomers across the four preceding generations. Although the goal in publishing the *observationes*, as Pomata analyzes it, was "collective empiricism," a shared body of knowledge that helped the community function, she also notes that *observationes* comes to represent "a specific product of just as specific an author/observer. It was, in fact, a deliberate effort to stamp observation with the mark of an author, and a model author at that" (p. 50).

Essential to the activity in question are noticing and recording, making detailed note of the features of a case, and acknowledging any variations on all relevant dimensions of the particular features that distinguish one situation from another. The detailing of variation is of obvious necessity to any painter of portraits or landscapes, any photographer, or naturalist discriminating sounds of birds in discovery of a new species. Importantly, the state of attention is included in defining the activity of observation and in rendering its epistemic status. Observing in this context is making note of variations with *great attentiveness*, what Pomata calls "quasi-religious care" (p. 52). In the same volume, Daston (2011) emphasizes the focus on particular events witnessed directly, personally, by a named author, and the creation of a community who collected observations into a relevant resource for shared purposes. Observations are the observations of *someone, a person*. In the identification of the record with the particular observer – in the researcher as an instrument, the reliability of the record is rooted in this instrument. Some instruments are better than others, as are some targets for observation: "[Observatores] do not amass their materials cursorily and, so to speak, by chance, without discriminating between authors, like the lexicrygraphs do. Observatores, in contrast ... collect their observationes from things most carefully read and considered" (Mario Niolio, 1535, quoted in Pomata, 2011).

Thus in addition to meticulous attention to detail and careful recording, observing required a proclivity to compare one's own records with those documented in received accounts – a willingness to question authority, we might say. An implication is that some persons are better at making observations than are others. It is not clear whether the difference in observational aptitude is a difference due to personal characteristics, disposition, temperament, or physical or intellectual capacities; however, there is *likewise* a clear implication that observational skills can be developed and refined with practice, for which reason the model or exemplar observations are used for the purposes of training.

Daston's scholarship reveals that by the eighteenth century, the general importance of observation to the advancement of knowledge across disciplines and interests was more widely celebrated. Naturalist Charles Bonnet wrote to a colleague that "the spirit of observation is the universal spirit of the arts and the sciences" (quoted in Daston, 2011, p. 81). As one example of this shared basis of arts and science, the ability to discern subtle differences in color and shading was of fundamental importance not only to the painter, but to the physician noticing a slight change of pallor as an indication of jaundice. The joint root of observation and observance is also consistent during this period with an all absorbing commitment to the practice of observation as a "way of life," one giving rise to emotional raptures and camaraderie with those of like mind.

By the eighteenth century, several observations of human nature became available, and philosophical reflection thereon seems to be closely linked to the idea of observation in its extensions to the realm of mental life (Hartley, 2013/1749), including aesthetics (Kant, 1960/1764). Interesting, however, is Kant's explicit distinction of the "eye of the observer" from that of the philosopher, suggesting "observer" as a kind of position taken on a subject matter rather than an abiding identity. Moreover, he equates observation with a casting of the eye, a deliberate activity employed toward a specified end, and involving a kind of case analysis:

> The various feelings of enjoyment or of displeasure rest not so much upon the nature of the external things that arouse them as upon each person's disposition to be moved by these to pleasure or pain ... The field of *observation* of these peculiarities of human nature extends very wide, and still conceals a rich source for discoveries that are just as pleasurable as they are instructive. For the present I shall cast my gaze upon only a few places that seem particularly exceptional in this area, and even upon these more with the eye of an observer than of a philosopher.
> (Kant, *Observations on the Feeling of the Beautiful and Sublime*, Section One, 1960/1764, p. 45)

Not only does the characterization of observation as absorption and commitment depart markedly from the view of observation as a detached, value neutral, or collective process, but the idea of dedication to observation as a way of life is testament to the holistic, integrative nature of the activity. For naturalists, at least, Enlightenment observation was "first and foremost an *exercise of attention*" (Daston, 2011, p. 99; emphasis added). Naturalist Jean Senebier published an essay titled *L'art d'observer* (1775), which proclaimed that "attention alone renders the observer master of the subjects he studies, in uniting all forces of his soul, in making him carefully discard all that could distract him, and in regarding the object as the only one that exists for it at the moment" (quoted in Daston, 2011, p. 99). Were we to import a label from our own time to depict the quality, we might characterize observation in this "important sense" as something like a form of mindfulness, or rather, we might construe mindfulness as integrally involved in observation in any domain. The products of this activity, collections of "observations" on topics in various domains of interest are owned as the work of a particular observer; they are the observations of someone, yet offered as considered and informative reflections intended to contribute to collective knowledge. The insights, though reflective of their subjective viewpoints, were held to be important and instructive for communal instruction. There was value in what was observed; it was held to be instructive to others if the observations proceeded from a reliable source – an observer, a person, whose observation could be trusted. On the other hand, Bacon, at least, sounded caution against the unchallenged acceptance of some received points of view, unexamined traditions of thought that impede understanding the properties, qualities, or propensities of nature:

> There are many ancient and received traditions *and observations* touching the sympathy and antipathy of plants: for some will thrive best growing near others, which they impute to sympathy, and some worse, which they impute to antipathy ... But these are idle and ignorant contexts and forsake the true indication of the causes.
> (Bacon, *Sylva Sylvarum*, Century I, 179; emphasis mine)

Bacon's cautionary note is a reminder of the various and perhaps compound meanings associated with observation at the time of his writing, a time characterized by transforming attitudes toward the ancient traditions and the wisdom bequeathed, especially in relation to nature. During this time too, the conceptual relation between observation and experiment underwent a series of changes, complicating the meaning and significance of both of these (see, e.g., Daston, 2011).

OBSERVATION AND INTELLECTUAL "PASSION"

What is most striking from the brief historical overview of older meanings of observation is the way in which observation was understood to be an exercise of persons, an originative act highlighting features of a situation. As a product, it reflected the endeavor of a unique being with unique interests and talents. Case analysis is an important example of what is produced through observation understood in this sense, as a kind of "noticing." Case studies are valued for their attention to specific details, especially discerning the particular features or details that distinguish one situation from another, enabling general features to be discerned through inductive analysis, providing a foundation for sometimes groundbreaking theory (e.g., Breuer & Freud, 1957/1895). Yet Hacking, as noted, regards "being observant" in the important sense he describes to extend to the act of noticing anomalies, a slight difference in pattern or design, making the observation in the sense of "noticing" details indispensable to experimentation as well as case study analysis.

Conceptualizing observation as an act of persons enables insight into its connection with other dimensions of being. An important connection is emotion, or in Polanyi's term, "passion." Although Polanyi does not focus on observational acts as such, he discusses what we have been calling "noticing" in a roundabout way in the context of his discussion of discovery, in conveying the importance of emotional investment or "passion" as this manifests in engagement and attention to specific objects and not others, for which reason he calls intellectual passion an "indispensable element" and an "essential quality" of scientific practice and eventual insight:[3] "What is this quality? Passions charge objects with emotions, making them repulsive or attractive, positive passions affirm that something is precious" (1974/1958, p. 134). What bears stressing here is Polanyi's desire to show a clear line of direction from passion to "objective" discovery, highlighting that the scientist's interest and personal involvement with what is studied is vital to the work of science, including though not limited to observation.[4]

CONCLUSION

The activity of observation or *observing*, despite a controversial and complicated history, may be understood as important to any method in the ordinary but highly important sense of "noticing" differences and discriminating particular features that distinguish one thing or situation from

[3] Polanyi's description of the function of passion in observation is similar here to Kohler's depiction of the function of "values" in science (1938).
[4] Polanyi's analysis of "personal" knowledge and its relation to establishing objectivity extends into all contexts or phases of science practice, including justificatory practices.

another. This is a basic cognitive ability to be sure, long acknowledged as related to intelligence, reliant on "tacit" or unverbalized processes, and one more keenly developed in certain persons. However, conceptualized as an activity, "observing" becomes amenable to cultivation, development, encouragement, with skill and practice, and is integrally related to other skills such as facility with language. Observing is marked with the style and stamp of the person, but must be made accessible to others, bringing the topic of observation into close relation with questions of representation, communication, even rhetoric – all forms of sense-making, as we shall discuss in the chapter to follow. The topic is also deeply, if not inextricably, connected with that of perspective, and the possibility of cultivating perspective-taking as an ability, the topic of Chapter 5.

4

Imaginative Sense-Making

One has but to open the door to any forces of exhibition at all worthy of the name in order to see the imaging and qualifying agency called at once into play and put on its mettle.

(Henry James, 2009/1904, p. lix)

The previous chapter emphasized that the nature and function of observation ("observing") as an epistemic activity of persons has been largely overlooked within psychology in recent decades, and suggested senses in which observing remains centrally important to any psychological inquiry. This chapter examines the related category of activity I will call *imaginative sense-making*, a term used to convey two ideas: first, that observing always involves active meaning-making; and second, that imagination is involved in transferring meaning into new domains, forging new combinations, and organizing observations into models – all activities that are centrally important to conceptual innovation, including innovation in psychological science.

SENSE-MAKING

As earlier noted, the idea that observations must be distinguished from the meaning made of them has been historically important to the project of objectivity, to the goal of eliminating bias and rendering scientific observation accountable. Yet many cognitive scientists and philosophers of science attest that observation cannot occur independently of meaning. Bartlett said it succinctly: "nobody has ever been able to find any case of the human use of evidence which does not include characters that run beyond what is directly what is observed by the senses ... people *think* whenever they *do* anything at all with evidence" (Bartlett, 1951, quoted in Bruner, 1973/1957,

p. 218). Moreover, for science it is not enough to make private meaning of observation. Observation must be shared and communicated, enabling others to make similar meaning of it or take the meaning into new directions.

Sense-making is a term used in reference to the active constructing, construing that constitutes "doing" something with observation, with evidence (De Jaeger & Di Paulo, 2007) and the acts of rendering observations intelligible to others (Gooding, 1990). It is a term that conveys both the bodily (sense perception) and the collective dimensions of meaning-making ("makes sense" both to oneself and to others). Such active "going beyond" sensory information to make meaningful experience at every turn is the very nature of thought, as Bruner (1973/1957), James (2007/1890), Kelly (1955), and others have emphasized, in cornerstone texts of early cognitive theory. That language itself structures observers' experience, providing the categories of meaning through which experience, reflection, and communication are even possible, is emphasized within the linguistic or discursive turn in philosophy (e.g., Austin, 1962; Wittgenstein, 1953), symbolic interactionism (Mead, 1934), social constructionism (Gergen, 1985), and related frameworks, calling into question the very intelligibility of the idea of "bare facts."

Bruner's description of "acts of meaning" remains vital even at our new frontier, for he affirms a transactional framework for understanding meaning that jointly positions agentive/intentional and cultural/collective dimensions of sense-making: to understand human beings we must allow that intentional states structure their acts and experiences, but we must also understand how "the form of these intentional states is realized only through participation in the symbolic of the culture," making it simultaneously a personal and a collective process (Bruner, 1990, p. 33). Bruner's account is highly compatible with what I have been framing as a person-centered framework for understanding psychological science. Sense-making is the activity of an embodied and storied agent who is ensconced, embedded, or situated in systems of personal and cultural meaning that both provide its conditions of possibility and "position" one in relation to others (Harré, 2012). It is activity that is as necessary to experience and survival as to any "higher" epistemic aim.

The term *sense-making* is so encompassing that we must work to parse out a particular sense of it that helps to clarify its relation to generative science. In this vein, *sense-making* serves as an umbrella term for the various and sometimes interlacing forms of activity designed to organize observations for various purposes in the science and practice of psychology: developing taxonomies, making predictions, summarizing themes in an assessment battery, or communicating an insight relevant to a pattern in a client's childhood experience. The degree of rigor and complexity and the goal toward which the sense-making is directed distinguish the everyday sense-making necessary for survival from the forms of sense-making engaged in interpreting test results or constructing mathematical models of physical or social systems, yet there is a similar effort to answer the questions "what might this be," "what can I expect of it," and "why might it be relevant?" fundamental to all forms and contexts of sense-making. Colleagues and I defined sense-making in relation to science practice as "shorthand for the continual efforts of any person to sort, understand, plan, and evaluate experiences of any kind, thereby giving them meaning" (Osbeck et al., 2011, p. 29). We aligned our understanding with that of organizational theorist Weick (1995), who emphasized that sense-making is both social and cognitive, collective and personal.

The inseparability of observation from sense-making in practice has proven important to various critical projects in philosophy and psychology as a basis for calling into question the legitimacy of the epistemic foundation claimed for empirical (evidenced based) science (Hanson, 1958; Feyerabend, 1975; Gergen, 1985). I wish to exploit the inseparability for another purpose here, namely to draw attention to ways the interrelation of observation and sense-making functions as an epistemic affordance for psychological science. Active sense-making, the activity of sense-*makers* (acting persons), that is, is precisely what enables theoretical advance. In other words, the active, creative nature of conceptualization is instrumental to and indispensable for scientific progress, including any progress that has been made in psychology. In keeping with the general thesis of this volume, it is an important epistemic priority to better understand the means by which this active sense-making is accomplished in psychological science, and in better understanding it, to underscore its value.

CONCEPTUAL CHANGE AND ANALOGY

Within philosophy of science, the active nature of thought and its relation to generative theory is discussed under the broad problem of *conceptual change* in science, on which there is a vast and complex literature (e.g., see Nersessian, 2008, chapter 1; Tweney, 1985). We can hardly scratch the surface of this topic here, but it is important to point out that there is little attention to the problem of conceptual change as it impacts the advancement of theory in psychology, other than in discussions of the relevance of paradigm shifts (Kuhn, 1962) as a basis for understanding psychological systems, most notably in relation to the "cognitive revolution" (Baars, 1986). The topic harbors a range of issues that are underemphasized, even ignored, in standard accounts of psychological methods. And as is the case for "observation," a closer look at the means by which transformative thought is made possible through imaginative sense-making reveals important connections between the "activities" fundamental to arts and sciences.

I will illustrate the importance of the topic of conceptual change or transfer with reference to a familiar psychological experiment.

CASE EXAMPLE: THE COGNITIVE MAP

A fascinating example of creative sense-making may be found in the set of experiments linked with the eventual undoing of the behaviorist stronghold and the promotion of a representational, conceptual, cognitive view of learning that allowed, even embraced, the inclusion of hypothetical entities in psychological explanation. Tolman's *Cognitive Maps in Rats and Men* (1948) demonstrates remarkable sense-making strategies and inimitable personal style, even as it reveals a set of deeply held values, both "personal" and reflective of its cultural situation. Tolman begins with reference to a set of then-recent studies of spatial learning, which typically positioned a hungry rat at the entrance to a maze with food waiting at the other end. The rat was allowed to wander freely, and the trial was repeated every twenty-four hours to maximum performance (i.e., progression through maze in a few seconds with no blind-alley entrances). Acknowledging that "all students agree as to the facts" but disagree on "theory and explanation" (p. 189), Tolman opposed the interpretation of stimulus–response (S–R) psychologists who sought to explain improvement in task performance in terms of strengthened stimulus–response connections, with the rat seen as "helplessly responding to a succession of external stimuli – sights, sounds, smells, pressures, etc. impinging upon his external sense organs – plus internal stimuli coming from the viscera and from the skeletal muscles" (Tolman, 1948, p. 189). By contrast, Tolman aligned himself with "field theorists" who regard the relevant brain processes as "more complicated, more patterned and often, pragmatically speaking, more autonomous than do the stimulus–response psychologists" with a nervous system that is "surprisingly selective as to which of these stimuli it will let in at any given time" (Tolman, 1948, p. 192).

Tolman's alliance with field theory represents a conceptual transfer in its own right, given that Lewin articulated his conception of the field in the context of social and organizational psychology (Lewin, 1946), specifically in reference to a model whereby "the person and his environment have to be considered as *one* constellation of interdependent factors" (Lewin, 1946, pp. 239–240). Thus Tolman (along with some contemporaries) adopted a concept from organizational psychology in the service of explanation of a single rat's demonstrated learning curve. Lewin's own application of field theory to social/organizational behavior itself reflects a transfer from the context of physical science (the electromagnetism field). The original "field" metaphor itself entails a transfer from the contexts of everyday life.[1]

The field is not Tolman's only generative metaphor. His best-known concept, the cognitive map, entails a transfer from the context of navigation to the context of rat special learning. Moreover, in this paper Tolman invokes the map not only as a static entity but as a "map control room," implying an active, dynamical system of communicative agents – a functioning "organization" localized in a single rat–environment system:

> Secondly, we assert that the central office itself is *far more like a map control room than it is like an old-fashioned telephone exchange.* The stimuli, which are allowed in, are not connected by just simple one-to-one switches to the outgoing responses. Rather, the incoming impulses are usually worked over and elaborated in the central control room into a tentative, cognitive-like map of the environment. And it is this tentative map, indicating routes and paths and environmental relationships, which finally determines what responses, if any, the animal will finally release.   (Tolman, 1948, p. 193; emphasis mine)

The analogy of human map-making to rat learning supported the five categories of experiment Tolman and his associates designed: latent learning, vicarious trial and error, searching for the stimulus, hypothesis, and spatial orientation tasks, and made possible the collection of new forms of data and an interpretation converging around the conditions that favor formation of broad or narrow maps. We would not say that Tolman claims to discover "maps" qua maps in rats, any more than he claims to discover a literal room. His innovation is clearly his insight that in its complexity, neural organization is *like* a map *control room*; the emphasis is on the function, not the literal features of maps. In the control room the incoming material is "worked over and elaborated,"

---

[1] See Lakoff & Johnson, 2003, Chapter 6, on the origin of "visual field."

suggesting a systemic and even agentive operation. Thus the metaphor also invokes anthropomorphism.[2]

Important for our purposes is to note the deliberate, perhaps even playful, importation of a concept from another domain. Tolman deliberately employs a metaphor and develops its theoretical affordances for conceptualizing unseen psychological processes, suggesting that the map control room provides the most fitting depiction of the intricacy of neural activity and the complex dimensionality of the organism environment system. The map control room is superior to the metaphor of a telephone exchange to which Tolman contrasts it. The new metaphor thus functions to open new trajectories of research, new discoveries, new knowledge, not only for Tolman himself but for generations of researchers influenced by him. The metaphor has *epistemic value* for psychological research; it is not merely a poetic enhancement or literary flourish, though it is obvious that its use reflects Tolman's theoretical alliances, and his description reflects his particular sensibility or "style." Importantly too, the specific metaphor chosen is a culturally and historically situated artifact. The term *map control room* had special potency in a postwar United States characterized by extraordinary innovations in navigational and computational technologies and cross-disciplinary advancements in communication theory.[3]

The metaphorical status of "map" is yet more obvious in Tolman's concluding remarks, when it becomes clear that it enables him to extend the implications of single-rat learning to the far more complex and challenging domain of human interaction, what he calls the "great God-given maze which is our human world" (p. 208). That is, Tolman uses the map metaphor to make an additional transfer – a transfer from the relatively contained context of rat spatial learning to the murky context of human social relations, invoking the labyrinthine character of the latter. He stretches the metaphor beyond anything trite or expected, equating "wide maps" with rationality and social tolerance, and narrow maps with "blind and unintelligent and in the end desperately dangerous hates of outsiders." With almost evangelical fervor, he acknowledges that his only answer to the perils of the world (and psychology!) is "to preach again the virtues of reason – of, that is, broad cognitive maps" (p. 208), with conviction of the broader impact

[2] For a discussion of how anthropomorphism can acquire functional significance in scientific contexts, see Osbeck & Nersessian, 2013.

[3] Smith (1990) analyzes cultural and personal context for Tolman's map metaphor within a broader discussion of postbehaviorism and its metaphors.

of the map metaphor for addressing problems of profound human significance, certainly relevant but not limited to the cultural/historical context in which he addresses them. Smith asserts that Tolman's metaphors "appear to have played a crucial role in formulating the world view from which his testable ideas arouse and within which his testable ideas arose and in which they found their true significance" (1990, p. 246).

GOING BEYOND: NEW COMBINATION, RECONFIGURATION, AND SURPRISE

During the same period in which Tolman was exploiting the affordances of map metaphors, Jerome Bruner devoted considerable thought to the question of "going beyond" the information given. Bruner, of course, acknowledged that meaning structures sensory experience with influences of expectation, language, norms, and interpretive acts, by which perception itself becomes an act of meaning-making. Much of Bruner's attention was to basic cognitive operations of categorization and their adaptive significance, the relation of meaning to perception, attitude, and direction of thought in everyday cognition. Yet he also made instructive remarks on the nature of scientific thinking in the context of this framing of "going beyond." His views on science converge around the idea that "the temper of modern science" (in contrast with that of the Newtonian period) is "nominalistic" (rather than "realistic"). Science is characterized by an emphasis on the scientist's active construction of models and theories "that have a value in going beyond the information given" (1973/1957, p. 233).

Bruner's views on creative thinking connected the writer, artist, and scientist at the level of desire to create – what we might characterize as a shared sense of the value of creating. He depicted the creative act as "an act of the whole man," and expressed his conviction that value lies in the act (activity), precisely because of its wholeness, rather than in the particular product created by means of the activity (1973/1962, p. 209). Although he distinguished several forms of creative thinking, he noted that they all originate in *combinatorial activity*, defined as "a placing of things in new perspectives" (p. 211): "Creative products have this power of reordering experience and thought in their image" (Bruner, 1973/1962, p. 212). Bruner considered the possibility that creativity should be understood as fundamentally metaphorical, given that metaphor functions to connect divergent domains of experience – things previously kept apart: "Experience in literal terms is a categorizing, a playing in a syntax of contexts. Metaphoric combination leaps beyond systemic placement, explores connections that before were unexpected" (p. 210), engendering not only effectiveness but new experience.

Though he referenced Poincaré (2001a/1913), Bruner found little available research or theory on the combinatorial acts central to the creative process prior to the time of his writing, and called for psychology to seek a more precise understanding of their nature. Without diminishing his contribution, we might note that there are historical precedents that Bruner does not cite. Thagard (2014) pointed to similar emphases in eighteenth-century philosophy; Hadamard noted important nineteenth-century contributions emphasizing the combinatorial principle in relation to the psychology of discovery (1945). As we acknowledged in the case of Tolman's maps, *metaphor* is both reflective of combinatory processes and a resource for new ways of thinking. As expressed by Lakoff and Johnson: "cross-domain correlations in our experience ... give rise to perceived similarities between the two domains within the metaphor... as when a love relationship, conceived of metaphorically as a partnership, goes awry when responsibilities and benefits are not shared equally" (Lakoff & Johnson, 2003, p. 245).

Thagard's focus is combinatorial neural representations (linguistic, propositional, sensory) that operate according to reliable and discernible mechanisms, by means of which the creative process is demystified on his account. Of interest is Thagard's own use of metaphor to support his preference for a theory of recursive binding, built around a mechanism of convolution rather than synchronization of neural firing:

> Convolution of representations is something like braiding hair, which typically combines three separate strands. The strands are woven together into a single strand which looks different from the original hair, but which can eventually be unbraided to return the hair to its original shape. Similarly, convolution takes two or more vectors and "braids" them into a new vector that can operate as a whole and can, when desired, be unbraided into the vectors that compose it (Thagard, 2014, p. 292).

Here is use of a metaphor to clarify the nature of the creative combinatorial process and its significance, expressing the idea that the strands of hair become something that seem different when woven, but remain able to be separated back to the original state. The use of metaphor in this case represents an effort to explicate and clarify rather than develop new directions of inquiry. Yet in this case, too, the metaphor has epistemic value. Explication and clarification are important epistemically in their own right; the metaphor aids in rendering a theoretical position accessible, facilitating understanding, which enables other agents to build upon it for research and scholarly purposes of their own.

The root meaning of metaphor is to "transfer a word from one place to another," implying that it "drives the statement in unexpected directions"[4] (Donoghue, 2014, p. 1), for which reason metaphor has received extensive philosophical attention in relation to rhetoric since Aristotle. In suggesting that creativity might be understood as principally metaphorical, does Bruner mean to suggest that all creative thinking has a linguistic or rhetorical form, or does he mean to imply that a broader understanding of metaphor might be required? Certainly Bruner regarded language, rhetoric, and narrative as central to meaning-making (see Brockmeier, 2009; Sarbin, 1986, 1993). But in this earlier stage of his writing, at least, Bruner's inclusion of *formal* (mathematical) relations in his discussion of creative transfer, and his connection of formal transfer with metaphorical transfer, casts doubt on the idea that he viewed metaphor as merely linguistic or rhetorical.

METAPHOR IN SCIENCE

There is a broad literature on the importance of metaphor in science, including in psychology, although historically its role in theorizing has been controversial. Metaphorical theories including Lewin's "field" theory were especially suspect in logical positivist circles from roughly 1920 to 1955, when rigorous theory was defined as *literal* theory with clear specification of intervening stimulus and response variables and no "surplus of meaning" (Hoffman, 1980, p. 394). In the context of the logical positivist commitment to literal language, the aversion to metaphor may stem from the assumption that metaphor involves imagination, opening the door to bias: According to Gergen, "[w]hereas literal language has been viewed as directly representing the objects to which it refers, and thus as being essentially 'true to fact,' metaphoric language has been said to be suffused with imagination, to be purely figurative, and to be exaggerated" (1990, p. 268). On critical view, metaphors do not correspond literally to facts,

---

[4] Important to note is that *simile* implies only likeness and does not function to move and reconfigure in the way accomplished by metaphor (Donoghue, 2014).

thus at the least lack predictive value, and at worst may mislead or invite spurious conception of phenomena.

The suspicion cast toward metaphor in the early twentieth century is traceable to the emphasis on direct sensory observation and effort to derive descriptive statements that correspond directly to sensation (without theoretical embellishment, preserving, as discussed, the idea of distinct "observations"). Lakoff and Johnson analyze historically deeper forms of resistance to metaphor, attributing it to fallacies traceable at least to Aristotle: that metaphor is a merely linguistic, not conceptual phenomenon – "a matter of words"; that metaphor is based on similarity; that concepts are literal and representational, not metaphorical; and that rational thought is independent of our bodily nature and experience (2007, p. 244). Of these, Lakoff and Johnson claim, the greatest obstacle has been the emphasis on metaphor as a literary device, a matter of style and persuasive function, which impedes recognition of the *conceptual* nature of metaphor (p. 245), its profound relation to the structure of reasoning itself, including scientific reasoning.

As we discussed in the previous chapter, the mid-twentieth century saw philosophical critique of the insistence on literal description, even of the possibility of literal description (Wittgenstein, 1953). As the insights of Tolman and Bruner testify, the mid-century also bore witness to remarkable advances in cognitive theory, and with these advances came increased affirmation of the value of metaphor in scientific theorizing. We might call this a recognition of the importance of metaphor in scientific sense-making, especially as a strategy for conveying hidden or tacit features of a phenomenon. Thus Max Black (1955) depicted metaphors as cognitively necessary, suggesting that they serve an indispensable role in scientific reasoning because they effectively reconfigure the phenomenon of interest conceptually and in so doing induce similarities that are grasped only through the metaphor. Metaphors were thus seen to have their own "logic" beyond the grasp or reach of logical positivism (Nemetz, 1958); they were recognized for their importance not only to deepen understanding but to facilitate new questions (Hoffman, 1980). Two important psychological works expressing similar ideas during this period include Schön's *Displacement of Concepts* (1963) and Wheelwright's *Metaphor and Reality* (1962), which explored the implications for understanding not only how metaphor plays a fundamental role in thinking but how it functions in relation to the origin and treatment of clinical pathology.

METAPHORS AS ANALOGICAL MODELS

Later in the twentieth century, cognitive-experimental studies emphasized the status of metaphors as analogical models, meaning that they function to project the schema of one domain onto another and thereby provide an aid for understanding complex relations. This view finds root in the idea of analogy as a kind of "seeing" one phenomenon in terms of another (Polya, 1945). Discussions focused on the affordances of analogy for providing new ways of "talking": "Argument Is War" is one of the best known examples for Lakoff and Johnson, who note that "the vocabulary of war provides a systematic way of talking about the battling aspects of arguing ... e.g., attack a position, indefensible, strategy, new line of attack, win, gain ground, etc." (2003/1980, p. 8). To understand what is entailed in classifying metaphor as a form of analogical model, and how metaphor is conceptual, generative of new thinking, it is necessary to look at least briefly at the nature of analogy and its relation to innovative thought in scientific contexts – how it is used by acting persons. A host of important work on the nature of analogy in science and in cognitive development more generally may be found in cognitive studies of science dating from the 1970s, with detailed analysis of metaphor's conceptual affordances (e.g., Gentner, 1983; Hofstadter, 1995; Johnson-Laird, 1983; Vosniadou & Ortony, 1989). As one example, Gruber analyzed Darwin's notebooks to advance a view of how Darwin's "tree of knowledge" metaphor enabled new directions in his understanding (Gruber, 1974). Although distinctions between "structure-mapping" in scientific and literary domains were a focus in some of these efforts, there is more recent philosophical interest in exploring the realm of fiction as a basis for gleaning insights into the role of metaphor in thought more generally, including in scientific reasoning (e.g., Camp, 2009; Elgin, 2014). If anything, some recent analyses have even more strongly emphasized the fundamental role of analogical reasoning in all creative thought (e.g., Hofstadter & Sander, 2013).

Much earlier, the precise means by which analogy functions in the service of generative thought was addressed by Poincaré, who helped to clarify the sense and means by which conceptual transfer in the form of analogy is an aid to thought, including mathematical and scientific reasoning. Bruner, indeed, made reference to Poincaré in developing his idea of the combinatorial and metaphorical nature of creative reasoning, paraphrasing him as emphasizing the apprehension of combinations that "reveal to us unsuspected kinship between ... facts, long known, but wrongly believed to be strangers to one another" (2001b/1914, as quoted in Bruner, 1973/1962), a new ordering and arranging that brings new aspects into view, including elements internal to the situation (hence, formal).

Pertinent to the title of our present work, Poincaré comments on the function of metaphor in the volume of his writings translated as *The Value of Science* (Gould, 2001). In the following passage, analogy is a source of *constraint* on the set of all possibilities offered for generalization from particular results:

> In a word, to get the law from experiment, it is necessary to generalize; this is a necessity imposed upon the most circumspect observer. But how generalize? Every particular truth may evidently be extended in an infinity of ways. Among these thousand routes opening before us, it is necessary to make a choice, at least provisional; in this choice what shall guide us?
>
> *It can only be analogy* (Poincaré, 2001a/1913, p. 274; emphasis mine).

Poincaré follows this statement by acknowledging that appeal to analogy as that which guides extension of observation introduces a good deal of conceptual ambiguity: "But how vague is this word! Primitive man knew only crude analogies, those which strike the senses, those of colors or of sounds. He never would have dreamt of likening light to radiant heat" (p. 274). But Poincaré then speaks of "the true, profound analogies, those the eyes do not see but reason divines," of the "mathematical spirit" that finds them, a spirit that "distains matter to cling only to pure form" (p. 274). This spirit, however, bestows its gifts only with diligence and focus. He credits Maxwell's theoretical innovation in electromagnetism to being "steeped in the sense of mathematical symmetry" (p. 275), such that by "looking at" the equations "under a new bias," he "saw that the equations became more symmetrical when a term was added," though it was a term "too small to produce effects appreciable with the old methods" (p. 275). The idea that a new perspective on the equations (a new bias) was necessary to grasp the underlying structural similarities is an important aspect of what is conveyed here. The account of generalization as a process of selecting the most appropriate and best analogy is resonant with Polanyi, who asserts that comprehension is a "responsible act" that makes contact with a hidden reality (1974/1958, p. viii). Poincaré establishes "felt sense" (what we might call "aesthetic value") in his account of how even generalization from observation becomes possible. It is a felt sense of rightness, an irreducibly aesthetic sensitivity activated in reasoning that serves to guide the agentive choice that constitutes generalization.

Through analogical models, relations between phenomena with no apparent physical resemblance are made evident. In the case of structural or mathematical analogies, "the laws of one of these phenomena aid us to divine those of the other" (Poincaré, 2001a/1913, p. 276). Models do not merely serve to describe, to summarize existing states of affairs, they also move things forward, they enable us to go beyond, to "see" relations *differently*: "To sum up, the aim of mathematical physics is not only to facilitate for the physicist the numerical calculation of certain constants or the integration of certain differential equations. It is besides, it is above all, to reveal to him the hidden harmony of things in *making him see them in a new way*" (p. 276).

We may see, indeed, the possibility for analogy to open not only new directions of thought within a domain, but more provocatively, open new domains of inquiry, including new directions of scientific research and theory. In *Science and Method* (2001b/1914), Poincaré depicts astronomy itself as fundamentally based upon analogical model:

> Astronomy offers us magnificent spectacles, and raises tremendous pro-
> blems. We cannot dream of applying the experimental method to them
> directly; our laboratories are too small. But analogy with the phenomena
> which these laboratories enable us to reach may nevertheless serve as
> a guide to the astronomer. The Milky Way, for instance, is an assemblage
> of suns whose motions appear at first sight capricious. But might not this
> assemblage be compared with that of the molecules of a gas whose proper-
> ties we have learnt from the kinetic theory of gases? Thus then method of
> the physicist may come to the aid of the astronomer by a side-track.
>
> (p. 359)

In a statement that prefigures the contemporary naturalistic turn in science studies, Poincaré asserts that we by means of active observation of scientists at work will be better able to understand the precise nature of the means by which the scientist "selects" from among the infinite possibilities available for observation and analogical modeling. The importance of analogical models to the creation of new scientific concepts or novel application of existing concepts has indeed borne out in both historical and empirical studies of scientific practice in recent decades (e.g., Tweney, 1985; Nersessian, 2008). Perhaps most interesting for our purposes is Poincaré's suggestion that *psychologists* would do well to study scientific practice, to learn something about the nature of discovery by means of such observation.

ANALOGY, METAPHOR, AND PSYCHOLOGY

Analogy to other sciences is a highly relevant topic for psychology for several reasons. Empirical psychology is itself founded upon an analogy to physical science: it is through analogy to physical science that a scientific psychology was imagined and pursued, and through analogy to chemistry that the search for the elemental building blocks of consciousness was established. The analogy to physical science has also been the trigger for a stockpile of criticism that challenges the adequacy of a conceptual and methodological transfer between physical and human science. Psychology, like astronomy, "offers magnificent spectacles and raises tremendous problems," not least of which is the difficulty consciousness poses for "observation," as we discussed in the previous chapter. But by comparing the elements of consciousness to elementary units of matter, the method of physics (experimentation) "came to the aid" of the psychologist through analogy, and similarly by a sidetrack, opened a path to years of laboratory investigation and the creative adaptation of methods to suit the goal.[5] Note that by contrast, a different analogy, namely to ecological biology, may be seen in conjunction with functional psychology (Angell, 1907), and calls for a different level of analysis and a different set of methods, with different implications (Osbeck & Nersessian, 2013). We also noted in the previous chapter that Watson's declaration of behavior as the only legitimate data source for psychology is derived by means of analogical comparison to physical science, wherein rigor is rooted in the experimental setup rather than in the training and subjective readiness of the observer.

The analogy to natural sciences has played a formative role in psychology's development overall – its existence as a discipline, but we may identify other ways in which analogical models in general and metaphor in particular have contributed to the conception and execution of empirical projects in psychology. Many of these developments are analyzed in an excellent set of essays edited by David Leary (1990), who identifies metaphor as "not only a form of speech, but more fundamentally a form of *thought*, having basic epistemological function" (Leary, 1990, p. 1) with "all knowledge ultimately rooted" in it (p. 2). The essays analyze the specific directions psychological research has taken on the basis of metaphorical thinking that both afforded and constrained it. For example, Karl Pribram traces both implicit and explicit uses of metaphor to aid understanding of the intricacies and complexities of brain activity. Telecommunications has

---

[5] I do not downplay the points of critique aimed at structural psychology, only note the role played by analogy in its conception and execution.

provided the most important source of analogies, beginning with the incorporation of techniques for measuring signal patterns in energy impulses transmitted in a communication channel. We may also note the map control system earlier discussed, and eventually, of course, the transfer of computer technology and the computational metaphor, by means of which the brain is viewed as a computational system processing symbolic representations. For neuroscience, as Pribram explains, not only are metaphors used "repeatedly and fruitfully" in an effort to understand their data, but "the proper use of analogical reasoning sets in motion a self-reflective process by which, metaphorically speaking, brains come to understand themselves." Echoing Poincaré, Pribram notes that "only by the proper use of analogical reasoning can current limits of understanding be transcended" (Pribram, 1990, p. 79).

Some literature on metaphor emphasizes its role in the creation or construction of meaning through interaction (Black, 1962; Gergen, 1990). Metaphor on this view functions as "the chief vehicle through which we advance our understanding of social life" (Gergen, 1990, p. 267), for which reason the ethical dimensions of metaphor use in psychology become exceedingly important to explore. That is, what metaphors have problematic social or ethical implications, and how might this impact their selection and use in the service of theory? In Gergen's view, for example, metaphors related to mechanism are inherently problematic in theoretical accounts of human activity and interaction, a view later expressed by Smythe (1998) in the context of calling for renewed attention to "persons" in psychology. Gergen suggests that what is required is a set of alternatives to the metaphors of mechanization, alternatives that will advance understanding of human transformative possibility and meaning-making. There is no single set of metaphors that will accomplish this aim, and those that do may be found in unexpected corners. As noted earlier, Tolman's (1948) map metaphor offers affordances for expression of his social values, his hope for challenge and eventual remediation of problematic social attitudes through the affordances of the map metaphor, with "broad maps" the key to a more just and tolerant society (see also Smith, 1990).

ANALOGY, IMAGINATION, AND VISUALIZATION

Metaphor, as a linguistic phenomenon, is embedded in and reflective of its historical situation – the terms, concepts, and situations meaningful to persons in a given cultural setting (such as map control rooms, computers, mechanism). However, although relying on the conventions of language, and therefore in one sense a social or collective phenomenon, metaphors also draw on our embodiment – they stimulate or facilitate the imagination, frequently conjuring a corresponding image. We noted also Poincaré's appeal to felt sensitivities and aesthetic resonance as a guide to analogy choice. It seems most accurate to conceptualize metaphor and other analogical modes as social and embodied, collective and personal – products of acting persons.

A fascinating historical resource for exploring the imaginal dimensions of formal analogy is Hadamard's *The Mathematician's Mind: The Psychology of Invention in the Mathematical Field* (1945). In addition to underscoring the combinatorial function of creative and synthetic thinking by means of analogical reasoning, Hadamard imbues his analysis with reference to unconscious processing, unconscious cognition, which although "strictly speaking, a business of professional psychologists," he notes, "is so closely connected with my main subject that I cannot help dealing scantily with it" (p. 21). The act, the "leap" of insight in any domain, with leaps closely linked to the affordances of analogy, is preceded by "the necessary intervention of some previous mental process unknown to the inventor, in other terms, of an unconscious one" (p. 21).

Most interesting is Hadamard's view that the unconscious has a "manifold character," in the sense that "several and probably many things can and do occur in it simultaneously" by means of which the synthetic function of science, the insight attained by combinatorial activity, becomes possible. We might call this manifold character multiperspectival, informed by and active from multiple vantage points at any moment. The conscious ego, by contrast, "is unique" (p. 23), i.e., is singular in phenomenal point of view. That is, conscious awareness assumes by necessity a singular vantage point, engendering a sense that one is unable to escape it. We will discuss the topic of perspective in the following chapter and explore the implications as they relate to interdisciplinary collaboration.

Consistent with an acting person framework, Hadamard uses the language of *choice* to account for the processes entailed in generalization and problem-solving. The manifold nature of unconscious processes provides the basis of synthetic combinatorial acts but does not complete them; combinatorial acts are necessary but not sufficient: "It is obvious that this first process, this building up of numerous combinations, is only the beginning of creation; even, as we should say, preliminary to it . . . to create consists precisely in not making useless combinations and in examining only those which are useful and which are only a small minority. Invention is discernment, choice" (1945, p. 30). Hadamard references Poincaré repeatedly in developing this line, and shares the earlier theorist's view that what guides the choice are rules, but not in the sense of rules that can be explicitly described, much less followed like a recipe. Rather, rules have the nature of "emotional sensibility," "an affective element." The affect in question includes not only "the will of finding" but more importantly and profoundly, "the intervention of the sense of beauty playing its part as an indispensable means of finding" (p. 31). The magnificent term Hadamard uses for this sense is *scientific beauty* (p. 31). The heuristic required identifies as an *emotional sensibility* (citing Poincaré), suggesting that fruitful combinations are guided by and recognized in emotional sensibility (aesthetic values, we could say), in the feeling of harmony, proportion, beauty, or rightness of form. Emotional experience is accompanied and aided by what Bruner notes that physicists speak of as "physical intuition," the distinguishing mark of the good theorist, consisting in "a sense of what combinations are likely to have predictive effectiveness and which are absurd" (Bruner, 1973/1962, p. 211).

That the "felt sense" is accompanied by visual imagery of some kind in most if not all instances of productive problem-solving is an additional theme Hadamard develops and relates to his own experience, describing the images that accompany mathematical insights in his own case, but relating the experience of visual imagery to the nature of generative thinking more broadly. He acknowledges that the topic of visualization in problem-solving has a long history, being tied to the broader concept of image and imagination and its role in thought, whereby it may be found in various forms at least as far back as Aristotle.[6] Hadamard's own examples include the image of circles in relation to the idea of sets, the vague image of a line with numbers, or, in relation to the theorem "the sequel of prime numbers is unlimited," an image of "a point rather remote from a confused mass" (1945, p. 76). Although he acknowledges that there are individual differences in the extent to which persons, even mathematicians, think in and with pictures, he also asserts that such "strange and cloudy imagery" is necessary to problem-solving: "I need it in order to have a simultaneous view of all elements of the argument, to hold them together, to make a whole of them ... It does not inform me on any link of the argument (i.e., on any property of divisibility or primes); but it reminds me how these links are

---

[6] Note visual roots of "intuition," "insight," reflecting a metaphor of "intellectual vision" (Osbeck & Held, 2014).

to be brought together" (p. 77). He asserts, in fact, that "every mathematical research compels me to build such a schema" (p. 77).

The "embodied cognition" framework has recently engendered greater emphasis on the visualizing and affective aspects of metaphor, and the role of metaphor in emotional expression (e.g., Johnson, 2007). Karin Moser thus argued that metaphor is a holistic concept, and as a psychological object one that can be analyzed both quantitatively and qualitatively – how often it is used and how it functions in various linguistic contexts. For psychology, metaphor is an inherently cross-cutting unit of analysis, we might say, yet one underutilized and underappreciated by the discipline in the main, not only as a focus of study in its own right – that is, its relation to everyday life – but as a methodological tool for our science, a creative, culturally contextualized act that aids scientific reasoning and facilitates problem-solving. In considering metaphor as analogy, we need to do more than identify specific examples of metaphor that infiltrate psychology, interesting as this might be. There is also a need to understand how analogy contributes to new conceptualizations, opens a window to new lines of question and new forms of research. This is of course a topic within the broader literature on scientific creativity, far too vast to cover here. However, I wish to emphasize that a study of this literature brings to the fore the active nature of cognitive practices, including the intentional use of analogy on the part of research scientists in every specialty, including the physical sciences. My suggestion is simply that psychology stands to benefit from better understanding of the means by which scientific innovation incorporates analogy and metaphor, and how metaphor invokes visualization, conceptualization, and communication, and thus how these insights in turn might advance the projects and methods of psychological science.

There is an extensive body of theory and research on scientists' reasoning through analogical models. These accounts of science practice are positioned in contrast to received or traditional views of scientific reasoning as hypothetico-deductive or logic-based in nature; they instead regard active modeling and "model-based reasoning" practices as the signature of much research in the sciences, both in discovery and application (Cartwright, 1997; Giere, 1999; Hesse, 1963; Magnani, Nersessian, & Thagard, 1999; Nersessian, 1984, 1992, 1999, 2002). Nersessian's historical and ethnographic work on model-based reasoning and its relation to conceptual change is exemplary, as are the methods she uses to derive accounts of the reasoning process (detailed in Nersessian, 2008). She has analyzed historical records (correspondence, notebooks, drafts, marginalia), focusing in particular on Maxwell's reasoning in creating a mathematical representation of the electromagnetic field, to offer an account of how scientists generate and extend new concepts. She later launched a comprehensive multiyear ethnographic investigation of research practices in the interdisciplinary contexts of bioengineering labs. Without denying the sociocultural contributions to science practice (for example, she views laboratories as "evolving distributed cognitive systems"), Nersessian's account highlights the active nature of the researcher in "going beyond" the information given, as Bruner would say, in the continual activity of modeling and refining models, a practice that she identifies as "genuine" reasoning. Researchers in innovative contexts construct and use models continually, not as an "ancillary aid" but that which enables inference in relation to a phenomenon of interest. Models, according to her account, may be structural, functional, or behavioral *analogues* of target phenomena, constructed to "satisfy constraints" (spatial, temporal, functional, causal, categorical, or mathematical). Importantly, they are not mere copies of the phenomenon of interest but are "ampliative" (i.e., they go beyond, expand), and in this sense "can be creative" (p. 184). Important to emphasize here is the active nature of the modeling practices on the part of the researcher that contribute to conceptual innovation, whereby an initial "rudimentary understanding" is transformed into a model that can serve predictive purposes. Analogical and imagistic processes are among those involved in constructing models, and according to Nersessian's analysis, "An initial model is created through which the *problem solver attempts to combine and integrate* constraints from both domains" (emphasis mine), "guided always by the goals of the problem solver, which are themselves reflective of the historical and current goals of the scientific community of practice to which the researcher intends to contribute" (Nersessian, 2008, p. 184).

IMAGINATIVE SENSE-MAKING IN ART AND SCIENCE

The ontological status of theoretical models used in scientific reasoning is a problem of considerable philosophical interest. That is, questions surround the nature of the organized "representation" researchers use to generate and support inferences concerning a target phenomenon. As we can see in Hadamard's account, a central question concerns the extent and nature of the "imaginal," a focus that brings questions concerning modeling practices into a nexus of relation with questions concerning the role of imagination in other domains of representation such as portraiture, landscape, and literary characterizations (see, for example, Frigg & Hunter,

2010; Toon, 2012). The set of questions concerning the extent to which models constitute forms of "fiction," even imaginal constructions that enable predictions that must then be subjected to verification and test, is part of a broader opening on the part of the philosophy of science community to a reexamination of the importance of imagination to scientific reasoning, to seek a deeper understanding of the "scientific imagination" and the relation of the imagination to knowledge. Relevant foci include not only modeling but thought experiments; analyses offer evidence and argument in support of a view of imagination as a necessary foundation of groundbreaking, frontier science in physical science and biology (Frappier, Meynell, & Brown, 2012; Gendler, 2004; Kind, 2016; McAllister, 2012; Stuart, 2018), including accounts of the means by which imagination provides access to universals, given that they are not accessible to the senses (Elgin, 2014). Thought experiment used in the service of evaluating models also underscores that imagination is not relevant only to the discovery phase of scientific reasoning. Analyses of imagination in philosophy do not downplay the complexity of the task of understanding and defining imagination, or of providing a taxonomy of its varieties and its relation to other cognitive kinds. Moreover, it is important to recognize that the important issues concern not only linguistic and mathematical forms of analogical model but visual and physical models, invoking materiality and embodiment in profound ways that make clear, for example, complex dimensions of epistemic work accomplished by "image" (see Stafford, 2001).

There is a great wealth of literature to mine, classic and contemporary, that bears on the role of imagination in science. I must simply assert that psychology's projects are not served by ignoring or resisting it. My small purpose is only to point to the need to make understanding the role of imagination in science an epistemic priority on the part of the psychological community, and, further, to emphasize that through such exploration traditional assumptions concerning demarcation between the categories of activity fundamental to arts and sciences break apart. This acknowledgment, though simple, requires a fundamental shift in attitude, even in disciplinary identity, in how we understand scientific practice. There are long-standing resistances at play, resistances that are not easily overcome. Daston (1998) depicted a "fear and loathing" of imagination on the part of scientists themselves and in the common public conception of what constitutes adequate science. Daston's historical analysis locates the reactionary stance toward imagination, the resistance to acknowledging its contribution to the generation of scientific theory, to a growing conviction of bifurcation between the projects of arts and sciences erupting most forcefully in the nineteenth century, and on her view, related to loosening conventions surrounding representational practices in art: "The causes lay in new views of the artistic imagination as freed from all constraints of reason and nature, and in a new polarity between objectivity and subjectivity" (p. 88).

Given the rootedness of psychology's epistemic aspirations in the period from which the perceived art and science polarity derives, it can be little surprising that emphasis on imagination is not commonly found in connection with description of psychological methods, nor even in relation to the epistemic goals of psychology as an academic discipline. Imagination is not adequately *valued*, not prioritized, not cultivated on the part of the psychological community. The devaluing of the imaginal dimensions of psychological science has implications for the education and training of psychologists, and it sets limits on the scope and reach of psychology as a discipline, preventing or at least discouraging systematic consideration of what is *possible* for human beings, and for the discipline that attempts to understand and help them.

QUALIFICATIONS AND ADDENDUMS

I do not represent this brief overview of issues related to imaginative sense-making as a review of the literature on scientific creativity, much less creativity in general. Key work on scientific reasoning has offered analysis of personal and system factors that contribute to scientific productivity and genuine innovation (Simonton, 2004), and has analyzed in detail the nature of scientific reasoning (Feist, 2008); contemporary work on creative insight analyzes the neural grounding of the acts (e.g., Kounios & Beeman, 2015). I have, instead, been concerned with the implications that follow from an acting person framework, wherein all scientific reasoning is both embodied and culturally embedded. I have suggested that imaginative sense-making, in particular that which makes use of metaphor and analogical models, constitutes one centrally important activity deserving of greater understanding and emphasis for its role in psychological theorizing.

It is important to note several points here. First, the idea that imagination contributes to scientific reasoning is not one that escapes skeptical reception and critique in contemporary discourse; indeed deep concerns are expressed about admitting appeals to imagination into even accounts of discovery (e.g., Matravers, 2010). Second, it is important to note that a claim that imagination is involved in scientific reasoning is hardly equivalent to a claim that scientific reasoning is reducible to imagination, or that imagination is all that is important to understand. Rather, the task is to understand how imagination interacts with processes of evaluation, how evaluation functions to hone and refine models to which imagination has contributed. Hadamard (1945) depicts the process as one in which consciousness intervenes, being necessary for the obvious expression of insights into sharable, communicable form (beyond inchoate feelings of relation or pictorial experience). He further specifies two *activities* that must accompany inspiration, "to verify" or test (to ascertain that one has not been "deceived" by unconscious combinations) and "to precise" them – in verbal or mathematical form. Nersessian's research suggests that model-based reasoning occurs in "cycles of construction, simulation, evaluation, and adaptation of models that serve as interim interpretations of the target phenomenon," a process she labels "bootstrapping" (2008, p. 185). Evaluation consists in making deliberate comparison between the features of the model and the target, in line with the problem to be solved and the specific goals of the researcher; adjustments to models are made on the basis of the comparison and subjected to further evaluation in a continuous loop. It is important, in sum, to regard imaginative sense-making as necessary but not sufficient, a component (though indispensable) of the coordinated set of acts that integrate to establish a foundation for making claims that can be evaluated, with adjustments.

Third, there is hefty challenge in attempting to understand how imagination contributes to science, yet at the same time to take seriously the way in which knowledge is embedded in normative systems that structure the sense-making processes through which imagination operates (Bruner, 1990). That is, how do we reconcile the need to prioritize imagination in science with the cautions long sounded against "spectator" views of science (Dewey, 1938), the private language argument (Wittgenstein, 1953), and the general problem of making genuinely novel scientific insight accessible to others and therefore in important senses shared, contributing to a collective empiricism from which others can draw and benefit? In earlier work, Nersessian and I aligned our analysis of practicing bioengineering scientists with accounts of science practice that recognize that neither purely cognitive nor purely sociocultural accounts of science practice do justice to its intricacies as practiced, and have taken steps to illustrate the integration of personal and sociocultural dimensions by analyzing the language, gestures, and shared forms of representation as these intertwine with the personal history and goals of the researcher in addition to the goals of the laboratory as a system and the broader cultural frameworks of scientific normativity in which they operate, what we called the "enactment of models" (Osbeck & Nersessian, 2006). In the subsequent chapter, I will examine how perspective-taking, aided by imagination, can work in the service of facilitating collaborative problem-solving and hybrid conceptualizations within interdisciplinary contexts.

5

Perspective-Taking

To that then I settled – to the question of giving it all, the whole situation surrounding her, but of giving it only through the occasions and connexions [sic] of her proximity and her attention; only as it might pass before her and

appeal to her, as it might touch her and affect her, for better or worse, for perceptive gain or perceptive loss: so that we fellow witnesses . . . should feel in strong possession of it.
(Henry James, 1934/1909, p. 145)

We can hope, too, for more flexibility in the capacity of inquirers to enrich their vision by trying on the spectacles of their neighbors.
(Sigmund Koch, 1993, p. 902)

The previous chapter explored various activities under the category of imaginative sense-making and focused especially on the active construction and use of analogical models, including metaphor. In this chapter, the emphasis is on the activity of perspective-taking, by which I refer to the deliberate practice of adopting different points of view, different vantage points in relation to a phenomenon of interest. I will admit at the onset that "perspective" is conceptually ambiguous, almost as ambiguous as the concept of "identity" with which it intertwines. Moreover, there are at least three aspects, categories, or senses of perspective that are important to distinguish: scientific and disciplinary perspective, paradigmatic perspective within discipline, and personal/cultural perspective. Although there are areas of overlap between them, I will discuss the three senses separately, and then return to a discussion of perspective-taking more generally in support of the aims of the chapter. I will argue that the activity of perspective-taking is important to cultivate in the interest of interdisciplinary collaboration, and that it also facilitates flexibility and problem-solving within disciplines. As is the case for observing and imaginative sense-making, perspective-taking is of value across the arts and sciences. In framing perspective-taking as an activity, I mean to emphasize that it can be cultivated at the communal level (the community of psychologists) in such a way that facilitates or enhances its instantiation at the personal level (in the researcher), which will in turn impact the projects of the community.

First, however, a few words about controversies surrounding the topic of "perspectival knowledge" are necessary to situate our discussion of how different senses of perspective are to be distinguished here as epistemically important.

OVERVIEW: PERSPECTIVAL KNOWLEDGE

To speak of "perspective" in any context other than the strictly visual is to speak metaphorically, though visual metaphors in epistemology are common. "Perspective" within the context of epistemological discourse implies a limited, bounded, or partial "view" of the world, or of some phenomenon within it. In this way an appeal to perspective, especially in the context of a claim that knowledge itself is perspectival, contrasts with traditional conceptions of objectivity, with the goal of providing a single, accurate description of "the way the world is" (Putnam, 1981, p. 49), a "fact" that can stand as a permanent addition to the knowledge pool.

It is within the context of the so-called "science wars" that pit "naïve realists" or "objectivists" against constructivists or constructionists (frequently assumed to be tinged with a form of relativism) that the term *perspective* can become a divisive slogan. A claim that multiple perspectives on a phenomenon increase objectivity (Harding, 2015) can be conflated with a claim that there are multiple competing truths, with no means of distinguishing between them or judging their merits other than through social convention. Such an idea is obviously incompatible with the search for a single universally true view of the world obtained through scientific discovery (e.g., Proctor & Capaldi, 2006). From this position, it is a short step to a project of attempting to dismantle the epistemic authority of science: "to the extent that the genesis of knowledge can be traced to communal life, the sciences cease to be the arbiters of the real" (Gergen, 2001, p. ix). Fears are roused because perspective can take on a connotation of bare assertion or opinion, reflecting political aspiration or wishful thinking, leaving power to determine the accepted narrative. In an era in which the issues of spin and bias are never far from discussions of journalistic or political integrity, fears relating to the idea of perspectival knowledge are particularly intense, and the implications especially serious. In the realm of education, we must consider what is at stake in implying that the perspective (if defined as opinion) of a researcher steeped in years of inquiry into a problem is no more authoritative than that of a first-year college student who offers opinion without having read the assigned text. Moreover, there are lines of implication from the epistemic to the moral realm. If any given locus of meaning-making is impermeable to an external judgment that might label its actions inappropriate or immoral, the grounds of possibility of moral action are at the least called into question, as is the basis upon which legislative action may be justified.

These concerns aside, we should note that it is hardly accurate to move from acknowledgment that aspects of knowledge are in important ways socially constructed to a conclusion that such knowledge is utterly lacking in epistemic or ethical constraints. Moreover, a line between social construction and pluralism is not directly drawn, in either direction. Constructionism and pluralism are distinct both historically and conceptually, and there are differing forms of both. There are highly sophisticated arguments in favor of both ontological and epistemological pluralism in philosophy of science that frequently pass under the radar of much of the psychological community (Kellert, Longino, & Waters, 2006; Harding, 2105). Moreover, there are differing versions of social construction and versions of relativism (see Harré & Krausz, 1995), with nuanced conceptual models of learning and knowledge construction as dynamical, interactive phenomena, and of linguistic, cultural, and historical constraints on the possibility of universal or even widely general knowledge. That political values infiltrate the dialogue is an obvious aside, yet positions on perspectivism (or social constructionism or pluralism) do not line up cleanly with conservative and liberal political values. It is true that during the 1960s countercultural revolutions, challenges to the idea of hegemonic, universal truth and method were embraced by those with commitment to upheaving the status quo and in the name of social justice. Yet more recently, the repudiation of claims to "alternative facts" and a pro-science agenda are common among those with progressive political views, with recognition of the need for public education in relation to issues of climate change, health care, and immigration policy.

After years in the company of theoretical psychologists, some of whom were pivotal to the rise of critical and constructionist positions in the discipline of psychology, I think that I have yet to meet anyone who genuinely believes that any given claim is indistinguishable in value from any other, though this is the position frequently attributed to those who acknowledge the importance of perspective. The more typical focus is on the legitimate range of methods used for psychological inquiry, with the altogether appropriate view that methods used to investigate psychological phenomena should follow from assumptions made concerning the nature of the phenomena and the questions posed in relation to them. This is closely accompanied by conviction that researchers have both an ethical and epistemological duty to reflect on the assumptions, commitments, and values they are bringing to a given research endeavor. As discussed in Chapter 2, values seem to direct many decisions made under the heading of methods, and values intermingle with group identities. This is the reason for the admonition to be transparent in acknowledging the perspective from which one views psychology's goals and in which one's methods are grounded. Yet there is an unacknowledged drawback to the politics of paradigm commitment. It is undoubtedly important to be clear about one's starting point, yet if one cannot or is unwilling to transcend one's own values (and those of the group with which one identifies), one is locked within a particular way of viewing the world, of viewing the work of psychology. This "locking in" prohibits or at least discourages genuine collaboration both within discipline (with those who identify differently) and between disciplines, especially where normative influences and expectations may be less formalized. As Nersessian and I have noted elsewhere in relation to interdisciplinary science, in order for collaboration between opposing positions to be possible, one point of view cannot be ignored or disregarded; one set of values cannot be imposed on the other (Osbeck & Nersessian, 2017). Negotiation is required, and such negotiation is only aided by understanding, by arming oneself to the extent possible with both the conceptual tools and the values that accompany alternative points of view. It is for this reason that perspective-taking can be seen as an activity with considerable epistemic affordances, one that is in principle and practice valuable to psychological science.

Perspective, however, is like most important concepts, one with multiple senses and meanings that are frequently conflated or denied. It is important, then, as a starting point, that we distinguish several forms or senses of perspective and perspectivism: scientific and disciplinary perspectivism, perspectivism as related to theoretical paradigms within discipline, and perspectivism as it relates to social and cultural identity or group belonging not limited to discipline or paradigm. There are clear areas of overlap between the different senses, but to treat them monolithically is to invite additional muddle.

1. SCIENTIFIC AND DISCIPLINARY PERSPECTIVISM

Philosopher of science Ronald Giere outlined an approach he called *scientific perspectivism* (emphasis in the original) in order to distinguish it from what he considered to be looser forms. Scientific perspectivism so described does not "denigrate into a silly relativism," but is consistent with a practice-based view of science, one informed by actual scientific practices rather than an a priori, idealized representation of science. Scientific perspectivism recognizes that science practice, including observation, is always constrained along a set of dimensions, and such constraint or limitation is the essence of "perspective" on this view. The strongest claims one can make are always of a "qualified, conditional form," because constraints are imposed both by the instrument used for making observations and by models through which inquiry proceeds, both of which set limits on the data to be obtained and what directions of inference can be made legitimately (Giere, 2010, p. 13). Instruments in any science are perspectival in just the sense that they detect or record "a certain range of aspects of the environment" (p. 41) and ignore other aspects. They are limited to the detection of some form of information, at certain times, and for certain purposes, whether the instrument is a telescope, microscope, tachistoscope, or intelligence scale. The human visual system is itself a constraining instrument, capable of yielding only a partial view of any object in the visual field and providing different views as different vantage points are occupied for different purposes, at a given time.

Giere offers case analysis that includes the neuroimaging technology so important in contemporary psychological research. Extraordinary advances in imaging technology over the past two decades have driven psychological research in new directions and have established a new evidentiary hierarchy, corresponding to a popular view that neuroscience offers contact with the material reality of the brain, the kind of hard and firm knowledge sought by objective realists. But as Giere argues, images produced by imaging technologies are not direct views of the working brain. Rather they are "images as produced by CAT or FMRI and so forth," produced *from a certain perspective*, which means in this case that this specific set of images – snapshots – was obtained and not others (Giere, 2010, p. 57). Moreover, the perspectival nature of the produced images bears a close relation to the human purposes according to which they were obtained. The images produced reflect a choice of some parameters over others, or a choice of some combination of parameters, at some time interval, and so on. There are trade-offs and negotiations, such as between speed vs. sensitivity, with additional decisions made about how to process the images. There are, in short, many possibilities for neural images, corresponding to different investigative goals, different problems, different agendas, both at the level of a given researcher and the larger collaborative project of which she is a part, not to mention the broader investigative system in which the agenda is prioritized, and most likely, awarded compensation or funding. The various ways of obtaining and using images all have relative merits or drawbacks and are weighed by human agents in keeping with some purpose at hand. To say that the decisions are informed by researchers' purposes is not to claim that the decisions are arbitrary or baseless; however, purposes constrain the range of data obtained, and thus render them perspectival.

Science is perspectival not only because observation (observing) occurs by means of instruments that "interact only with restricted aspects of the world" (p. 59), but also because theoretical models impose constraints. Like Nersessian, Giere regards the construction and use of models as a principal epistemic activity for scientists, an activity that constitutes sense-making, we could say, and functions in the service of representing the aspect of the world the scientist(s) is attempting to understand. As representational efforts, models have much in common with maps. Like maps, models offer a partial view, and are constructed and used for a given purpose. Models are in this sense "interest-relative" on Giere's account. In the case of neuroimaging, Giere points to the task of "brain mapping" used in the earlier period, especially in relation to CAT and MRI technologies that produced representations of structural features of brains. In the case of functional imaging (FMRI), the "map" comparison is more metaphorical, yet it captures the partial, perspectival, and interest-relative features of the task of producing images that are consistent across technologies.

Perspectivity in Interdisciplinary Science

Interests, of course, are shared to varying degrees. There are group agendas – those of a research team, a laboratory, a professor and her students, a topical journal, a subfield, the broader discipline. Within groups of various sizes and at various levels, models are developed and used in dynamic interactions between researchers in accordance with joint agendas, with mutually agreed upon problems and sets of principles used to inform them (e.g., thermodynamics, relativity, natural selection). These shared aspects of modeling and other representational and reasoning practices render scientific problem-solving a system-level phenomenon in an important sense. Such systems are at once cognitive, material, and social and cannot be adequately accounted for through reductive accounts of any kind. In the case of neuroimaging: "An MRI facility, for example, can be thought of as a relatively localized, but still quite complex, cognitive system for producing images of human brains and other organs. ... the system becomes larger if one includes the scientists or medical specialists who use them" (Giere, 2010, p. 100). The particular working facility is comprised of persons in interaction with each other, the highly advanced equipment, devices, existing models, sanctioned methods of procedure, a base of converging theory, and often a set of shared values. Thus an important aspect of scientific "perspective" is the implication of a shared or communal vantage point, shared assumptions and traditions of practice. Shared features of perspective are reflective of not only micro-level social interactions (researcher to researcher interactions: between coworkers, a mentor and those mentored, a laboratory manager and laboratory assistants, etc.) or interactions within a laboratory or other practice group, but also the broader discipline within which one is working, as well as cultural norms, historical situations, social structures such as Western university science, capitalist economic structures, etc. This feature of science practice prompts Nersessian's term *cognitive-cultural system* in reference to a functioning research laboratory dedicated to addressing a set of problems in a given area of specialized practice (e.g., systems biology).

Relationships with other researchers impose additional constraining conditions on inquiry: Roles are assigned (e.g., lab manager, post-doctoral student participant, principal investigator). Each of these roles is performed within a system of constraints (and affordances) specific to it; and violation of role boundaries upsets the workings of the laboratory and thus the projects of any science. There are, moreover, relational structures in place established by the historical project of science itself, or the varieties of science that evolve in relation to new goals (Osbeck & Nersessian, 2017). Rules are established within a community toward specific shared and personally meaningful ends. Interpretations of data then function not only as cognitive frameworks, but as rules of production for the knowledge domain under consideration.

Instruments and rules for their use are often tied to and bound by specific disciplines. In one sense, then, disciplines can be considered to offer a specific perspective on any given subject matter or problem. Yet the idea that crossing boundaries or integrating disciplinary perspectives facilitates generative thinking is increasingly recognized, reflected in interdisciplinarity, itself depicted as an "emerging cognitive science" (Derry, Schunn, & Gernsbacher, 2014). Earlier, Bruner, who emphasized that the structure of creative thinking might be principally metaphorical, also suggested that progress in knowledge is likely to be found at the junctures of disciplines, in the boundary land between fields, or in willfully traversing the boundaries. This view is consistent with the conclusions of contemporary investigations of scientific progress over the past two decades: "[I]nterdisciplinary understanding (i.e., the ability to integrate knowledge from two or more disciplines to create products, solve problems, or produce explanations) has become a hallmark of contemporary knowledge production and a primary challenge for contemporary educators" (http://wwwp2.harvard.edu/Research/GoodworksIS.htm).

Interdisciplinary understanding, understood as a form of integration, is contingent upon interdisciplinary collaboration, the ideal of which "engages participants in collaborative dialog, including debate and conflict, which both transforms the understandings of individual participants and produces new knowledge, new solutions, and even new disciplines that would not be possible without such dialog" (Derry & Schunn, 2014, p. xiii). As interdisciplinary scholars and policy makers have argued, there is a need to better comprehend and promote the conditions that foster interdisciplinary collaboration. There is a substantial literature on this question, conferences devoted to collaborative science, new programs and academic specialties – a new industry, in short, dedicated to the pursuit of understanding and promoting interdisciplinary problem-solving.[1] A major line of argument used to promote research into examining the conditions of successful interdisciplinary research is that the potential for confronting human and national challenges lies in the creative possibility and multi-perspectival view that such research can provide, with disciplines representing different vantage points from which problems might be addressed. Thus, for example, in Nersessian's study of bioengineering as an emerging interdiscipline, through various collaborative practices between engineers

---

[1] Most of the effort is directed toward interdisciplinary science, with specification of conditions that affect issues of funding and institutional support, such as physical space for collaboration, academic leadership, the size and nature of the problem to be solved, sufficient numbers of adequately trained scientists, and related factors. [For overview, see National Academy of Sciences, National Academy of Engineering, and Institute of Medicine (2005). *Facilitating Interdisciplinary Research.* Washington, D.C.: The National Academies Press. https://doi.org/10.17226/11153.]

and biologists, the laboratory moves as a cognitive-cultural system toward production of "hybrid" researchers with expanded problem-solving potential (Nersessian, 2012).

Nersessian's analysis is especially relevant to the topic of frontier thinking because she targeted practice communities focused on innovation at the margins or boundaries of two or more disciplines (Nersessian, 2012; MacLeod & Nersessian, 2015; Osbeck et al., 2011). Her adoption of a distributed cognitive framework for conceptualizing scientific practice brings into focus the shared nature of epistemic perspective without reducing problem-solving to social interaction. Nersessian's more recent investigation compared two integrative systems biology labs dedicated to cutting edge applications in computational biology but with different organizational structures: one a purely computational lab that obtains biological data by means of external biosciences collaborators; the other containing its own wet lab for conducting biological experiments in the service of model building. In a recent paper, Nersessian and I introduced the term *epistemic identities*, in keeping with our analysis that perspective is an aspect of disciplinary identity, but also that identity (and thus perspective) occurs around epistemic task or method (Osbeck & Nersessian, 2017). That is, epistemic practices such as adopting a particular method or level of analysis (e.g., a reductionist vs. a systems *perspective*) reveal epistemic values; epistemic values, in turn, are instantiated in epistemic identities. We found that differences in identification as modelers or biologists accompanied differences in attitude toward what constitutes the goal or aim of research.

A surprising but consistent finding from this study was that interviews revealed researchers to speak of disciplinary backgrounds different from their own in ways that we found critical at times, even disparaging. Characterizations of one's own or others' practices were not neutral; there was not a sense that different methods or "epistemic tasks" are equally useful ways to pursue knowledge, even within a laboratory that shares the broader normative framework of Western science and the local problem agenda of that particular laboratory (e.g., the manufacturing of artificial blood vessels for implantation in the human body). Researchers from different disciplinary backgrounds or with different skill sets (experimentation or computational modeling) expressed differing views of what constituted the overarching goal within the interdisciplinary research context and also different ideas about what constitutes good science. The ways of talking about other researchers' methods sometimes displayed an implicit epistemic hierarchy, with some practices positioned as more consistent with the researcher's view of science. Often these ideas seemed on the surface even incompatible, expressive of differing sets of norms and values concerning what it means to be a good scientist or to bring the appropriate emphasis, resulting in differing perspectives on level of analysis or overall problem-solving aim (e.g., description vs. prediction).This was at times a source of conflict to be managed or reconciled in collaboration or in making the transition to a new "hybrid" disciplinary category: a "bioengineer," even when the larger goals of the laboratory were shared or collective.

As we describe in the paper, modelers that described experimental work as routine, that they saw as emphasizing memory over reasoning, depicted experimenters as unconcerned about dynamic interactions and lacking in the mathematical skill required for creative modeling. Conversely, we found that some experimentalists characterized modelers as unrealistic in focus, naïve about (biological) reality, wanting things that are not always possible, seeking data that are not available. Among the characterizations are that modelers are unconcerned with what is biologically possible, that they function at the level of ideals and possibilities and not at the level of the concrete demands of the experimental process. There were comments that modelers do not know how to ask the right questions, that they do not understand the complexity and delicacy of balance required for experimentation, that their outcomes may not be practical, and that their focus is on possibility and speculation over precision.

These findings initially led us to worry about negative impacts on the potential for fruitful collaboration. Yet among the most interesting aspects of the study was the reason we found to be hopeful that a researcher can learn, through effort and targeted educational experiences, to adopt epistemic perspectives different from her own, and further, that she can move back and forth between perspectives in accordance with the epistemic task at hand. This optimism is rooted in case study of two researchers from different disciplinary backgrounds as they evolved personally and conceptually in the new "hybrid" environment. This case study analysis followed interviews with researchers chronologically, using line-by-line interpretation to track changes in their description of experiences over time (Osbeck et al., 2011). From the case studies, two events stood out as especially salient to the possibility of cultivating epistemic perspective-taking. In one case, a modeler who had enrolled in a summer camp program designed to develop skill in experimentation expressed a sense of broadening her perspective through the experience, describing a sense of having been changed internally through the program. In the other, a biologist expressed greater appreciation for and understanding of the affordances of modeling after enrolling in an introductory biosystems modeling course designed to give biologists and modelers a "feel" for modeling systems. In both cases, researchers described the focused learning as provoking a kind of personal transformation, experienced as a newfound ability to incorporate the other epistemic perspective. Interviews also revealed that in both cases the broadened perspective resulted in the researcher reporting a sense of being more effective in her original task domain. The modeler expressed a sense that the experimental camp experience had enhanced her relation to modeling, and the experimenter expressed a sense that understanding the modeler's perspective enabled her to provide more helpful experimental data in collaborations with the modeling lab. The two researchers also expressed a newfound sense of being able to move back and forth between the perspective of experimenter and the perspective of the modeler as the particular task might require. Nersessian and I emphasized that these findings suggest the value of strategic learning experiences, formal and informal, for enhancing epistemic awareness and cultivating an epistemic identity that is more flexible and better adapted to the demands of interdisciplinary problem-solving. In turn, we suggested that this expanded perspective and more flexible epistemic identity might contribute to more effective collaborations, better reasoning, greater awareness of affordances of methods, and broader range of cognitive tools (Osbeck & Nersessian, 2017).

2. PERSPECTIVE AS PARADIGM

However, it is not always, or perhaps even usually, the case that a disciplinary identity yields a single epistemic perspective. I have stressed the pressing value, even urgency, of including psychological contributions to broad scale problem-solving agendas that require interdisciplinary cooperation. However, psychology does not offer a unified set of concepts or method – a single psychological perspective. Instead, psychology is itself multiperspectival, fragmented, and already inherently interdisciplinary given that its concepts, frameworks, and methods bear the marks of physical science, social science and humanities, and divergent philosophical traditions.

Thus there is a need for understanding the possibility of intradisciplinary perspective-taking that borrows from the insights obtained through the study of interdisciplinary settings. If greater problem-solving potential is claimed for interdisciplinary collaboration, it follows that greater problem-solving potential is also to be found in enhancing collaborative relation-ships between psychologists from different theoretical or methodological traditions within discipline. Perspective-taking within discipline will aid in fostering conversation and bringing divergent skills and concepts to work on challenges beyond the scope of any one specialty area or theoretical framework. In recent years, psychology has witnessed intensified efforts to develop cross-disciplinary (i.e., within psychology) programming at national and specialty conferences. At the level of method, the mainstream status and legitimacy of mixed-methods designs is testament to genuine movement across traditions and frameworks.

Nevertheless, there remains a good deal of misunderstanding, even suspicion, between psychologists from different methodological traditions, or between those who identify with the tradition or mainstream of psy-chology and those who adopt a critical, human science, or other alternative perspective. Some of the resistance reflects a broader view that it may be naïve or misguided to think such collaboration or even conceptual transfer between disciplinary traditions possible given the markedly different, even incompatible, bases from which they proceed (e.g., see Byford & Tileagă, 2014). The first and most obvious "cut" dividing psychologists, at least, is one between those who embrace a view that qualitative methods are on equal epistemic footing with traditional experimental and correlative methods and those who do not embrace this view, or indeed, who consider double blind experimental analysis to be the gold standard for any psy-chological research. Though I do not have access to interview data to compare psychologists to bioengineers, I have a good deal of anecdotal evidence from years of participation in professional organizations in psy-chology, and draw from informal conversations with colleagues on each side of this divide. On this basis I am convinced that the relation between quantitative and qualitative inquiry in psychology is *analogous* to an interdisciplinary science, in that different traditions of inquiry engage different concepts, frameworks, and methods – that their researchers bring different perspectives to psychological phenomena. I am also con-vinced that these differing perspectives, if combined productively, might yield greater and more creative problem-solving potential than any single tradition on its own. I do not think that what is required is simply a matter of mixing methods for the sake of mixing methods (any more than mixing disciplinary perspectives arbitrarily), but of genuinely valuing the affor-dances of different disciplinary and methodological traditions and bring-ing these into fresh combinatorial relations that generate new methods, concepts, and models appropriate to complex new social realities.

The trick, of course, is to do so without losing the variation and particularity inherent in each. But at the level of person – the psychological researcher – I envision the task as one of expanding or enlarging perspectives, incorporating them in the service of a personal transformation, akin to the transformations expressed by the bioengineer. Such transformation is a matter of enlarging our maps, to borrow Tolman's metaphor, or broadening our value systems, in the terms I have been using throughout this text. If such enlargement is made possible on the personal level, the transformation of persons may extend to disciplinary transformation such that the problem-solving potential of psychology is expanded.

I know full well, however, that a Pollyanna view of collaborative potential within psychology is likely to be met with objection in light of the fact that perspectives are rooted in paradigms that are fundamentally incompatible, even incommensurable. Epistemic and ontological and ethical concerns cannot be easily untethered; they are embedded in seemingly mundane disagreements concerning units of analysis, schemas of inference, number of participants, and even style and accessibility of communication. Therefore methodological differences that represent or follow from divergent conceptual paradigms may simply not lend themselves to integration, even in the service of the most worthy problem-solving goals.[2] Nevertheless, it is a great understatement to note that there is confusion attending the appeal to perspective in the sense of paradigm, and that paradigm is a concept that has been used loosely for a variety of academic purposes for over half a century, since it appeared in Kuhn's landmark account of the basis and impact of shifts in scientific thinking over a half century ago. We should also note the close relation to "standpoint theories," on which the literature is vast (Harding, 1986).

In part due to its proximity to the onset of paradigm controversies in psychology, one of the most helpful discussions of the attending controversies is found in *The Paradigm Dialog* (Guba, 1990a), a collection of papers intended to offer reflection on the directions taken up by social scientists in the wake of Kuhn's analysis of scientific progress. Guba's introductory remarks acknowledge that most persons are unable to clearly define *paradigm*, a situation he finds unsurprising in light of the diversity of ways Kuhn is said to have used the term across the body of his writings (citing Masterman, 1970). Nevertheless, there is a "common" or "generic" sense of paradigm: "a basic set of beliefs that guides action, whether of the

---

[2] The very idea that psychology should concern itself with addressing broad "problems" is not one shared or equally acknowledged across the community of psychologists.

everyday garden variety or action taken in connection with a disciplined inquiry" (Guba, 1990b, p. 17). The concern of the edited volume is with the role of paradigms in directing inquiry, especially in relation to ontological (the nature of the knowable), epistemological (the knower's relation to the known), and methodological questions. Answers to these questions are the "starting points or givens," providing a "roadmap" for specific practices and procedures (p. 18). Paradigms are not derived empirically, of course; they establish the conceptual grounds upon which empirical inquiry can be conducted – they are a nonempirical grounding for the empirical. Controversy surrounding paradigms centers on the idea that they are "options for inquiry" (Guba, 1990a, p. 9). The idea that there are options rather than one true way, one "scientific method," is difficult for many psychologists. Positivism is itself presented as a paradigm, one of the options from which one might choose, and like all other options, heaves with values that cannot be eliminated by any procedural means and which must be simply claimed or owned as a choice, a matter of faith and commitment.

The criteria that precisely qualify a paradigm as an "option for inquiry" is not a matter that has been determined to any level of agreement. Philosophical defenses of pluralism underscore the importance of multiple perspectives on complex questions, and the value of differing stances in dialogical relation, analogous to the optimal functioning of a democratic society. Yet note the emphasis on dialog and exchange rather than on a cacophony of divergent voices. Some means of limiting the number of legitimate options or, at the least, a strategy or defensible grounds for eliminating illegitimate options may be needed to foster genuine dialog, to enhance the potential for influence on the part of more alternative positions, just as a limited number of parties serve as organizing structures in a political system. Feyerabend acknowledges that any tradition (traditions being defined and distinguished in terms of "different internal structures," p. 20) exerts influence on more powerful traditions only by gaining in internal strength, such that the power relations between traditions attain more balance. Yet this poses a fundamental conflict related to community and freedom. On one hand, the hegemony of any single approach is to be avoided; on the other hand, it is not permissible to strike out on one's own, untethered to any recognizable tradition. So genuine options are few, determined by convention and consensus, and require that any researcher's insights fit within the recognizable contours of an identifiable paradigm, determining the unit of analysis from which to theorize, the specific set of procedures to follow, and the end or goal of the inquiry as study of that particular kind (e.g., positivist, phenomenological, discourse analytic, constructivist). It is not surprising that one of the early criticisms of the paradigm concept in relation to social theory focused on the idea that a paradigm – any paradigm – might be considered to have its own set of foundations, which creates a set of binding obligations to constrain inquiry, but simply in different ways of being binding, or different sorts of binds (Lincoln, 1990). Among the questions is whether the assumption that there must be a paradigmatic structure to knowing, and the corresponding expectation to declare and adhere to paradigms according to the basic belief framework each upholds, might stifle the free play of inquiry, encouraging hegemonic and authoritative structures every bit as binding in their own ways as the positivism for which they were intended as alternatives (Osbeck, 2005).

The idea that paradigms are "options for inquiry" suggests that although the options are limited to existing paradigms, any researcher may freely select among those available, in line with values or interests, presumably. The idea of paradigms in this sense, as available options, as consciously and deliberately chosen to suit different purposes, diverges from Kuhn's original depiction of a communal phenomenon operating implicitly to influence observation and theory construction on the part of a broad scientific community in its specific historical situation. Moreover, the implication that there is genuine choice at the level of individual choosers, personal commitment to a paradigm, is difficult to square with the claims of paradigms that prioritize collective processes as the basis for meaning and moral reflection. Nevertheless, I use the term here to reflect the looser meaning it has acquired for many social scientists, that is as a theoretical or methodological option to which one demonstrates some commitment.

If choice among existing competing paradigm options is a matter of values, this returns us to the idea that methods, inasmuch as they reflect paradigms, constitute value systems. However, we also return to the problem that in practice, at least, paradigm choice (reflected in choice of methods) is shaped by power relations, for example in the fact that there are methods sanctioned by the majority in the field, which in turn has implications for the goal of obtaining an academic position or funding for a research project. That is, some persons will be empowered, and others will be disempowered by the adoption of any paradigm. Therefore choices made by researchers who are concerned with moral responsibility often reflect an intent to restore power balances through the selection of relatively underrepresented methods. This is, at least, an implicit message in some of the discourse surrounding the idea that paradigms represent options for inquiry. One may wonder, therefore, about the extent to which paradigm choice can represent a genuine choice at the level of the person (a personal choice, that is), if it has been predetermined that only some options are epistemically legitimate on one hand, or on the other hand, that only some paradigms are morally and ethically sound ones. The idea of positivism as one option among the many is revealing of the problem. If the tenets of positivism are so problematic that it must be replaced with more morally responsible options for inquiry, positivism does not constitute a genuine choice. Such a choice may be compared with that of a condemned property presented by a realtor as a housing option, presented alongside several other properties evaluated to offer safe and comfortable living quarters.

Guba's own goal is not so much to definitively argue for a particular paradigm, but to envision social theory as moving gradually toward superior and superordinate paradigms. This target minimizes some conceptual problems related to issues of "choice" among paradigms, but it does not eliminate the problem of the grounds upon which paradigms may be transposed, combined, grafted, or selectively bred, especially when their assumptions are incompatible, for example in the case of positivism and social constructionism. This question is related to the broader question of how any given paradigm might be evaluated in any way that transcends its own conceptual boundaries. Much has been written on these kinds of fundamental issues, and they interrelate with controversies surrounding method, raising questions about how journal submissions, presentations, and other scholarly contributions might be evaluated outside of the paradigm within which they were conceived and executed. These questions do not invite easy resolution but require ongoing conversation, and they are perhaps best regarded as a necessary fallout of the effort to broaden inquiry beyond the traditional confines of disciplinary contours.

Pragmatism and Perspective

An idea that occurred to some of us over the years was that paradigms might be compared and evaluated on the basis of some broadly pragmatic concern, an evaluative standard that enables paradigm "choice" yet remains relevant to the particular goals of the inquiry (Osbeck, 1993, 1995). The pragmatic framework, itself a paradigm of sorts in the loose sense of a set of beliefs to guide action, predates the paradigm controversy as it emerged historically. It represents an effort to offer a solution to the philosophical problems of its own day, to overcome false dichotomies pitting subject against object, and to foreground the fundamentally dynamic interaction of actor and world in the creation of knowledge. James's version of pragmatism is especially relevant to the goals of this chapter and book as a whole, because it provides a coherent means by which the project of choosing paradigms might be conceptually anchored, and a means by which perspective-taking can be construed as an activity to be cultivated in the service of transformative thought. My purpose here is certainly not to outline the whole of pragmatism or even the version James advances, but merely to feature aspects that bear directly on questions relevant to the issue of perspective-taking.

As is well known, the first articulations of what was to become identified as pragmatism were offered by Charles Sanders Peirce (1868), though James's book represents "the first self-conscious, thorough, and consistent attempt to explore the implications of pragmatist theory" (Vescio, 2003, p. viii). James begins his first essay in this work by aligning his views with those of "Mr. Chesterton," and affirming a person's "view of the universe" as the most important and interesting thing about a person. This view of the universe, James calls a philosophy, but not a "technical matter"; rather, it is "our more or less dumb sense of what life honestly and deeply means ... our individual way of just seeing the total push and pressures of the cosmos" (2003/1907, pp. 1–2).

In his introductory essay, at least, James connects perspective as "view of universe" (world view) to issues of personal style – to one's natural inclinations in thinking patterns, to temperament. He calls the history of philosophy "to a great extent ... a clash of human temperaments" (2003/1907, p. 3). Temperament, he asserts, is the basis of one's strongest biases, including the biases displayed by philosophers; it "loads the evidence" one way or another in any argument or demonstration. We trust our temperament, James notes, for which reason it serves as the rock-bottom foundation of our judgment, our perception, our theory of truth. We wish for a representation of the universe that suits our temperaments, and thus believe in those that do, finding those with opposing temperaments and consequent views of the world to be "out of key" (p. 3). The principal distinction James draws in this context is that between the "tough-minded" empiricist, who is skeptical and seeks facts, and the "tender-minded" rationalist, who is driven by idealism and principle. Empiricism and rationalism emerge as something like our contemporary notion of paradigms, at least as these have migrated into the realm of social theory. They are systems of beliefs that establish the basis for inquiry, epistemological positions with implications for methods; they constrain and structure inquiry; they attach to values. James admits that most of us lack a temperament so strongly contoured that judgments follow naturally and easily from it. Most of us are a mix, he says, with a "hankering for the good things on both sides of the line" (2003/1907, p. 6), and therefore easily swayed by the whims and methods of the day, or caught up in the eloquence of those we find impressive. Nevertheless, what has driven thought forward is that some persons do see things in a unique way and feel dissatisfied with opposing visions. On the other hand, the problem with such strength or directedness of vision is that it can blind us to other perspectives and thus limit our view.

What James depicts is a kind of whole person blend of embodiment and social influence that impacts our view of the world and everything in it, which is operative in the everyday life of just plain folks and in the professional lives of philosophers and scientists. The natural, everyday rootedness of our world view gives rise to the parallel idea that we must choose sides and defend them. It is deeply ingrained, including in academic circles, for which reason there is identity congregation around theories and paradigms. Broad acceptance of pragmatism itself on the part of the academic community would require a change at the level of temperament, James notes, and on this point, he displays characteristic pessimism, though he envisions pragmatism as a corrective to the shortcomings that accompany a rigid defense of one's preferred way of thinking at any cost.

Because beliefs connect to action, James sees the salient question to be one of whether beliefs adhere to satisfying or productive actions, which may include coherence with existing theory. As a *method*, pragmatism aims at providing a reasonable basis for evaluating "options for inquiry" to carry the theme of choosing between paradigms. Pragmatism is also depicted as merely an attitude, a looking forward rather than looking back, toward likely outcomes, fruits. In this depiction it is clear that the pragmatic method makes use of active imagination. It requires that we occupy possible or likely positions corresponding to theoretical alternatives, and requires evaluation of their likely outcomes, but from the point of view of the perspective taken, in keeping with the values and goals of that vantage point, that is, imagining where the assumptions are likely to lead. Although James connects the pragmatic method to the goals of empiricism, it is an empiricism informed by thought experiment and other richly imaginative exercises. As an example, James references Locke's discussion of personal identity: "'Suppose,'" he [Locke] says, "'one to think of himself to be the same soul that once was Nestor or Thersites. Can he think their actions his own any more than the actions of any other man that ever existed?'" (2003/1907, p. 40). And James offers his own exercise: "Imagine, in fact, the entire contents of the world to be irrevocably given. Imagine it to end this very moment, and to have no future . . . then let the pragmatist be asked to choose concepts" (p. 42). The pragmatic method is contrasted with "resting on principles" or imposing a world view without considera- tion of its effects. Theories themselves are "instruments, not answers to enigmas in which we can now rest" (2003/1907, p. 23).

If theories are instruments, they impose constraints on observation; they are inherently perspectival in the sense earlier discussed (Giere, 2010). They are used by persons for purposes, purposes that at once bear a relation to the goals of the practice community (shared expectations of psycholo- gists in a given specialty area) as well as to the personal goals of the researcher (a research agenda, relation to one's life's work, values). They reveal a relation to prior learning yet are not fixed and static. In this sense pragmatism does not seek to impose an external standard that is binding across beliefs systems: it is "oriented around possibility and promise" even as it holds all views to a general standard of bearing fruit (2003/1907, p. 23). "It appears less as a solution than as a program for more work" (p. 23).

The main point for the present purposes is that James's account of pragmatism offers a basis for comparing paradigmatic alternatives through imaginative sense-making, and with a focus on what is possible. As a method, it is deliberative activity in which any thinker can engage, which can involve purposeful occupation of different vantage points through intellective acts that include the engagement of supposition or the play of imagination. The "vital question for us all," he notes, is "what is the world going to be? What is life eventually to make of itself?" (2003/ 1907, p. 50).

However, evaluation of a theory or paradigm in terms of its likely outcomes requires intimate and substantial knowledge within that para- digm. A surface reading is not a legitimate basis for an out of hand dismissal and does not constitute grounds for choice, for such a surface familiarity cannot provide the basis for informed judgment of likely out- come. Evaluation of paradigms, like incorporation of multiple paradigms into a more superordinate "perspective," requires considerable effort and commitment to develop and "master" the tenets of an alternative para- digm, let alone multiple alternative paradigms. That is, superordinate perspective or flexible movement between paradigms, then, is made pos- sible only by means of a greater degree of rigor and accountability than that which is required by one alone. It is again a goal that may begin though the personal transformation and enlargement of those committed to intradisciplinary expertise, who may acquire through focused experiences the ability to utilize different instruments. Yet through such personal transformation we may see the potential for greater collaborative and problem-solving potential in the field (psychology) at large.

3. PERSPECTIVE AND IDENTITY

There is another sense of perspective-taking equally important to consider, yet one that presents even greater obstacles to precise and clear description. That is, perspective also corresponds to or follows from categories with which one identifies: sex (e.g., female), national or regional origin, religious affiliation, sexual orientation, gender, age, social class, and so on. It is tempting to refer to these as non-epistemic identities, to provide a contrast with the identities that relate to epistemic task or discipline, as discussed previously. However, these other categories also bear on epistemic concerns, as is clearly expressed in standpoint theories (Harding, 1986), so the label would not be adequate or accurate. That is, the relation is reciprocal: identification with groups provides perspective, and perspective is rooted in identifications of various kinds. Nevertheless there is no clear mapping of identity onto perspective. Perspective is not uniform across identification with groups. For example, the perspective of a person raised in a liberal college town in the 1990s may differ in important ways from that of a person who came of age in a rural village during the 1930s, despite a shared ethnic identity. Moreover, few, if any persons identify exclusively with a single group. Identities interweave in complex networks as they are enacted and lived; and personal identity is rooted in the configuration, the mosaic of group affiliations or estrangement from groups, as is expressed most powerfully in critical literature on intersectionality (e.g., Crenshaw, 1989).

There is a wealth of material from which to draw in relation to perspective-taking in this broader sense – decades of scholarship on identity and its implications in relation to questions of perspective as it impacts both knowledge and lived experience. To name but a few, contributions of feminist scholarship (Fox Keller, 1995; Haraway, 1988), indigenous psychologies (Kim, 1990; Sundararajan, 2015), critical psychology (Teo, 2015), narrative psychology (Freeman, 2014), and various forms of constructivism and constructionism prioritize the perspectival nature of understanding, both descriptively and proscriptively. Phenomenological psychology (Giorgi, 1970) and various traditions of qualitative methods aim precisely at providing systematic and thorough descriptions of parti-cipant experience. In giving voice to experience, these methods facilitate understanding of other identity perspectives, and often perspectives that are "other" than those of the main historical narrative represented in the discipline of psychology or in the culture at large. The effort to "give voice" to those whose voices have been unrepresented historically has been an important aspect of many qualitative research efforts over the past 30 years (see Wertz, 2014). Yet the association of perspective with societal position-ing, culture, or embodiment calls into question the means by which "perspective-taking" can be understood as a skill or activity to be culti-vated, thus calling into question the premise of this chapter.

For it is not easy to understand how we might occupy the lived per-spective of another person, to identify in ways that are outside of our experiential range. Here we encounter fundamental questions relating to the nature of social connectedness and social embeddedness of experience, with theoretical roots that extend backwards to some of the founding concerns of personality and developmental theory (Adler, 1964; Bowlby, 1988), and that predate the emergence of experimental psychology. Historical review by Coplan and Goldie (2011) asserts that *Einfühlung* was first used as a technical term by Theodor Lipps in 1874, not in relation to interpersonal understanding but in relation to a theory of aesthetics. It was used in designation of the means by which people directly experience objects and come to know the mental states of others, but it is regarded as the root of the word *empathy* (Coplan & Goldie, 2011). The closest meaning is "feeling into . . . a process of inner imitation or inner resonance that is based on a natural instinct and causes us to imitate the movements and expressions we perceive in physical and social objects" (Coplan & Goldie, 2011, p. xii). The concept was highly influential in philosophy, and the idea that the feelings of others are "given" through empathic responding came to serve as an important alternative to the analogical model of knowledge of mental states dominant in the early twentieth century, by which we know others' mental states by consulting our own and drawing inferences about others from what we find in ourselves. As "feeling into" became closely linked to understanding by Dilthey, Husserl, and others, it was central to the problems and methods of phenomenology and hermeneu-tics, and thus to the human science project as it emerged. Edith Stein's seminal work on empathy is especially important to understand, though her account of the nature of empathy diverged in important ways from that of Lipps (Stein, 1964/1917). Among Stein's emphases are the importance of seeing persons in their wholeness rather than as representatives of categories, and the possibility of expansion or transcendence of one's own constraints through empathic encounters, though her treatment of empathy and its relation to Husserl scholarship is far more nuanced and complex than this brief description can convey.[3] More recently, questions concerning social connectedness through empathy focus on empathic accuracy, the extent to which the ability to judge the feelings of others emerges as predictive of professional success and strong relationships, and overall psychological health (e.g., Gesn & Ickes, 1999). The neural basis for accuracy in empathic judgment is itself debated, with imitation of facial expression (e.g., Meltzoff, 2002) and more recently vocal communication (Kraus, 2017) identified as the basis of accurate empathic responding.

I mention these developments primarily in service of making the point that perspective-taking in the third sense under consideration is of a different nature than that of the other two senses discussed, and may require additional resources such as empathy, and with implications that extend beyond those of epistemic considerations. Perspective-taking in this sense has been discussed most frequently in the context of emphasizing the foundational relation of perspective-taking to moral reasoning – that is, the idea that moral reasoning and moral action are rooted in the ability to transcend one's own perspective and occupy that of another person (e.g., Ansbacher & Ansbacher, 1956; Hoffman, 2001). As one example, developmental theorist Ann Higgins connects skill in perspective-taking to moral education, following empirical investigation and analysis of Kohlberg's project to establish "just communities" in middle and high school settings (Power, Higgins, & Kohlberg, 1989). Higgins, like Kohlberg, considered moral education to be a necessary component of any school curriculum, especially during the crucial period of adolescence, when identity formation is a central developmental task (e.g., Erikson, 1968). Perspective-taking is key to the work of just communities on Higgins's account, not merely as a skill to be developed, but as an aspect of the developing self to be cultivated through focused experiences: "We believe that developing role-taking skills and perspective-taking influence students' views of themselves as moral beings and as moral agents, able to choose to act upon their ideas of what is right and good" (Higgins, 1991, p. 136). To the extent that qualitative research facilitates perspective-taking, not only developing skill but impacting the moral identity of researchers, we might note that an argument in favor of training in qualitative methods for all

---

[3] An excellent recent analysis by Kris McDaniel clarifies Stein's understanding of empathy and details of the debate with Lipps (McDaniel, 2014).

psychologists is that they might play a formative role in the moral development of the researcher.

Yet it would be mistaken to regard the perspective-taking most closely aligned with social identifications, including cultural, purely in terms of moral considerations, for what is at stake has epistemic dimensions as well. A compelling though still controversial question that spans cognitive science, philosophy of science, and anthropology concerns the extent to which there is diversity in cognitive processes across cultural contexts. That is, whether basic processes such as perception, categorization, attention, memory, and thinking show variation in form or style (how these processes occur) in addition to differences in content (what is perceived, remembered, believed). Claims in favor of "divergent cognition" fly in the face of the universalist pretensions of much cognitive research, whereby neural mechanisms are assumed to operate consistently across cultural boundaries. A recent review of the literature on cognitive diversity finds consistent, subtle though nontrivial differences in cognitive processing in accordance with cultural diversity (Bender & Beller, 2016). The authors account that different cultural tools and representational formats pose specific sets of constraints on cognitive processes. We have identified cultural variation as a different sense of "perspective" than that which Giere describes as scientific perspectivisim – perspective imposed by instrumentation and conceptual model. However, we can identify in the work on cognitive diversity across cultural identifications a similar emphasis on imposed constraint. Similarly, just as the ability to assume the perspective of modeling or engineering enhances epistemic power, perspective-taking across cultural identifications would effectively increase epistemic power. The most important implication that Bender and Beller identify from their review is the potential for greater understanding of cognitive diversity to enhance cognitive theory, to enable the refinement of existing models or the development of more adequate and inclusive models of cognitive phenomena as these phenomena are operative in the world (Bender & Beller, 2016). This view is consistent with what philosopher Sandra Harding identified as strong objectivity, referring to the view that diversity of viewpoint provides more comprehensive, thus ultimately more complete and accurate understanding of any phenomenon (Harding, 2015).

Cultivating Perspective-Taking

If perspective-taking enhances knowledge of complex phenomena, knowledge also enhances perspective-taking: the relation is reciprocal. Perspective-taking requires knowledge in addition to feeling, even in the case of perspective closely wedded to cultural or personal identity. An important point is that perspective-taking is aided by historical insight, historical consciousness. Perspective implicates power relations, power relations that have a history and analyzable effects in any present context. It is difficult if not impossible to occupy the perspective of any given cultural group without awareness of the historical conditions of advantage or disadvantage relative to other groups. Perspective-taking thus requires knowledge of the operation of these relations, of at least a broad sort in addition to knowledge of culture-specific representational style and content. Of course, the salience of historical situation is especially relevant in the case of systematically disadvantaged groups, wherein the historical positioning is central to the cultural representations that define and constrain the group's understandings of itself and other groups. For example, although historical knowledge of engineering practices is helpful and aids understanding of the "engineer's perspective," knowledge of history is indispensable for understanding perspectives associated with colonized or racial identities, including as these perspectives are enacted in science practices (e.g., Malone & Barbarino, 2009).

SUMMARY AND CONCLUSIONS

This chapter has examined several distinct senses of perspective as a means of emphasizing the epistemic importance of perspective-taking as an activity more generally. As should be evident, problems with arguments for and against the perspectival nature of knowledge stem at least in part from the insufficient distinction between the senses of perspective implied. On the other hand, perspective-taking of any of these varieties may contribute to enhanced understanding of psychological phenomena by providing multiple viewpoints and levels of analysis, leading to a more comprehensive account.

Moreover, despite differences between various senses of perspective, it is also possible to draw several points of emphasis that emerge by means of looking at all senses as a set, and thus to consider what is involved in the activity of *perspective-taking*, defined as a purposeful attempt to transcend a given vantage point, whether disciplinary, paradigmatic, or identity related, and to occupy another perspective to the extent possible. Such perspective-taking is necessary, I suggest, to problem-focused efforts, especially for problems of marked complexity. I emphasize "attempt," and "to the extent possible," because of course one is never able to genuinely transcend one's own stance; moreover, the stance may be altered in the act of attempting to transcend it. Nevertheless, it is also not the case that perspective is categorical in nature, that we are hopelessly encased in our own viewpoint and unable to expand or enlarge it, or unable to move back and forth between differing perspectives (e.g., even a reductive or a systems point of view) in the service of a problem-solving goal. Although perspectives are merged with values and commitments, even matters of faith, problem-solving is not helped by an unwillingness to understand other values and other ways of viewing the situation under consideration, or from the vantage point of different stakeholders. For example, recent standoffs within the psychological community (e.g., over methods, practice guidelines) do *not* reflect a problem-focused orientation.

I have tried to emphasize that perspective-taking increases opportunities for creative problem-solving and facilitates more comprehensive knowledge. Perspective-taking does not require that all perspectives must be accepted uncritically or as equal in relevance or value. Analysis as determined by epistemic, pragmatic, or ethical values is always required on both personal and collective levels. Nevertheless, the ability to engage in perspective-taking in each of the senses discussed in this chapter is essential to the goals of interdisciplinary collaboration and the ability to engage in new forms of problem-solving.

Two additional points of emphasis are needed. First, perspective-taking is a whole-person activity, engaging knowledge, imaginative projection, and emotion at a minimum. Second, perspective-taking requires effort and commitment. It often demands focused experiential learning (e.g., the modeling "camp"); education and fact gathering to understand differences in content, style, and values; and learning new "languages," either in a literal sense or in the sense of understanding the concepts, models, and values of another disciplinary position or methodological paradigm. It requires listening, reflexive examination of one's own biases and assumptions, and considerable motivation for expansion. In short, the activity of perspective-taking does not occur automatically but must be cultivated. To be cultivated, it must be supported. Its value must be appreciated and prioritized, affirmed and encouraged in a broader epistemic community.

6

Conclusion

Knowledge or science, as a work of art, like any other work of art, confers upon things traits and potentialities which did not previously belong to them.
(Dewey, 2008/1925, p. 285)

I would like to suggest that it is in the working out of conflict and coalition within the set of identities that compose the person that one finds the source of many of the richest and most surprising combinations. It is not merely the artist and the writer, but the inventor, too, who is the beneficiary.
(Bruner, 1973/1962, p. 216)

[t]he act has its way of abiding and showing and testifying, and so, among our innumerable acts, are no arbitrary, no senseless separations.
(Henry James, 2009/1909, p. ix)

Twenty years ago, William Smythe's introduction to a collection of essays titled *Toward a Psychology of Persons* attested to psychology's historical avoidance of "the person," an avoidance fortified by two opposing trends: on one hand, explanation directed at the level of biological and computational mechanisms, and on the other hand, extreme renditions of social and cultural constructionism for which subjective experience and agency receive little attention, and are at the least downplayed. Lost, on Smythe's account, was the "middle ground" of integration, a domain of persons. In the two decades that followed, some opening to persons and a person-centered psychology is evident, both in theoretical analysis (Bergner, 2017; Fisher, 2017; Lamiell, 2009; Martin & Bickhard, 2013; Martin, Sugarman, & Hickenbottom, 2010) and in empirical research designated as "person-centered," intended to be multidimensional, holistic, and temporally focused, in contrast with variable-based analysis (e.g., Ciarrochi et al., 2017). In both of these cases, there is recognition that "persons" imply special forms of analysis to adequately represent their complexity.

In the spirit of these openings, this book represents an attempt to foreground the person in psychology, but with a focus on the personhood of the researcher, and to consider what this focus implies for both the conception and practice of psychological science. The focus on the psychological scientist as person addresses a similar middle ground, or a similar gap, in the domain of science studies, which have largely addressed cognitive or social dimensions of science practice, contributing to what has been termed a cognitive–social divide by several scholars (Longino, 2002; Nersessian, 2005). In the activity of persons, the coordination of cognitive/rational and social/cultural processes is implicit, as are myriad marks of uniqueness, particularity, style, and whatever normative frameworks are in place to direct and constrain.

A focus on persons and their activities in any domain also foregrounds concerns with values. Values are an inescapable dimension of all activity in which persons engage, including the simple and complex activities that constitute scientific practice. The idea that "person" is a unique ontological kind has moral implications quickly following. Awareness of actions, ability to reflect on them, and ability to control or redirect them are the scaffolding or preconditions for responsible action and accountability.

To emphasize the personhood of the researcher does not mean that "evidence" is downplayed or unheeded. Rather, "researcher as person" serves as a reminder that evidence must be gathered, interpreted, compared, synthesized, weighed, and applied responsibly, by persons, in line with values. To view the "researcher as person" in the ideational context of "personalism" implies, additionally, that the values toward which these activities are directed will be those that emphasize the inherent dignity and worth of all persons, those that serve humanity as a whole and not the special interests of a subset.

Putting together the emphasis on activity and value in this volume, and considering the relevance of this amalgam for psychology, my concern has been with activities of special value, epistemic priorities. I have been especially engaged in exploring activities across methodological frameworks in psychology, at a level more fundamental than "method" or procedural specifics. First, I drew from a variety of sources, historical and contemporary, to suggest a sense of "observing" as an attentive "noticing" of detail – an awareness, especially, of differences between situations, an attention to pattern, and deviation from pattern. This is a more informal sense of observation, but it is consistent with the methods used by researchers who derive theory from studying children in naturalistic settings (e.g., Piaget, 1962, Vygotsky, 1978), and from participant observation methods common in cultural anthropology and its applications to psychology, in which the primary data are (along with interview content) detailed descriptions in the form of field notes (e.g., Atkinson & Hammersley, 1994; Emerson, Fretz, & Shaw, 2001). Yet it is also a sense of "observing" important to experimentation. Second, I suggested "imaginative sense-making" as an activity that moves theory forward into new domains. Metaphor, especially understood as a form of analogical model, provides what is perhaps the clearest case of this transformative function, and one that has been recognized as important in advancing psychological theory (Leary, 1990). I noted increasing recognition of the role of imagination for thought experiment and model construction as these activities contribute to conceptual change and the development of theory in all domains, including physical science. Finally, I suggested the importance of *perspective-taking,* defined as a deliberate effort to occupy a range of other vantage points, including disciplinary, theoretical, and identity-related perspectives. This list of activities is certainly not intended as exhaustive; it is rather more of a starting point in an exploration, a concerted effort to imagine what is implied for psychological science by a view of the psychological scientist as an engaged participant in a natural, technological, and social world she is charged with investigating, and whose problems are her own. I have been especially concerned with activities that will facilitate new directions of thought, interdisciplinary collaboration, complex modeling, and flexible problem-solving, because I believe these are increasing priorities in an era characterized by extreme and unpredictable global challenge.

I have not sought to distinguish natural science from human sciences for these purposes, but have been more concerned with questions that concern the connections between science and art, especially as these connections manifest themselves at the level of activity. For the three activities suggested take into account that to foreground the acting person is to recognize the *whole* person as engaged in problem-solving, which includes aspects the influence of which is not recognized or accounted for. Despite the fact that "agency" is emphasized as an aspect of persons, it should not be confused with the idea that insight can be willed into occurrence. Polanyi, D. L. Watson, and others who have emphasized the "personal" side of science have done so in recognition of nonconscious, unarticulated connections and reconfigurations that influence what is "seen," what sense is made of it, and what is prioritized, for which reason Polanyi refers to discovery as "a process of emergence rather than a feat of operative action" (Polanyi, 1964/1946, p. 33). Yet spontaneous reorganization and emergence rely on activities that are effortful, on what he acknowledged to be "an effort of mental concentration to evoke the knowledge of a real thing never seen before" (Polanyi, 1964/1946, p. 35). Effort and spontaneity work collaboratively, in loops extremely difficult to predict or even describe with accuracy. These features imbue scientific practice with an aspect of artfulness that should be no surprise, if acting persons direct their emotions and capacities in the direction of art or science as they are inclined by disposition, expectation, interest, and opportunity.

I have tried in this work to offer examples of specific connections between the arts and sciences at the level of activity, and to consider how these connections are revealed in the practice of psychology. However, because the connections are instantiated and revealed through the activity of persons, we are better served by specific exemplars (i.e., persons whose work illustrates the points of connection described in earlier chapters). Thus, to amplify points made earlier in this volume, I turn to illustration to examine the claims made in these chapters with reference to the specific case of William and Henry James.

ILLUSTRATION: WILLIAM AND HENRY JAMES

The James brothers provide fitting material for illustration for our purposes for a variety of reasons, but one of the most important is that they are both concerned with subject matter that is at least broadly psychological. They show keen interest in attending to fine-grained differentiations in experience, despite differences in their goals and methods. Although known for contributions in different academic arenas – general psychology and, later, philosophy in the case of William, and creative writing as well as literary criticism in the case of Henry, their intellectual practices demonstrate a remarkably similar blend of characteristics that, as they demonstrate, serve both scientific and literary purposes. We can discern Henry's psychological sophistication in his complex novels as well as in correspondence between the brothers published in a collection of letters (James, 2016), and in a detailed set of Henry's memoirs recently published as a set (edited by Horne, 2016). In turn, the artistry and poetic quality of William's writings have been noted by many authors (e.g., Leary, 1992).

Thirdly, the example of the James brothers also accentuates the social/ relational, cultural, and historical dimensions of "the acting person," providing an important counter to the idea that "person" implies a disconnected, disembodied, abstracted rational actor. William and Henry exhibited a close and intellectually enriching relationship with one another. The quality of that relationship as well as the unique education they enjoyed, their family values, atmosphere, and opportunities, and their father's friendships and collegial relations are helpful for understanding how "the person" must be understood as reflective of relationship systems of various levels. The particular historical and cultural moment they occupied is also necessary to an adequate understanding of person and that which is "personal."

I offered quotes from Henry James to correspond to each chapter. Here I can offer only a few illustrations of the ways in which the James brothers demonstrate observation, imaginative sense-making, and perspective-taking in ways that inform their different projects, and that are in the service of their different goals.

OBSERVATION

In Chapter 3, we noted that observation or "observing" was long regarded as the foundation of scientific discovery, the basis for generating data: in short, evidence. Yet "observing," in the sense of engaged attending and noticing, especially discriminating the fine details that differentiate one situation from another, is also essential to the work of any artistic form. In drawing attention to the observational skill that both William and Henry James exhibit in abundance, we must acknowledge the overlap between observation and expression – the ability to communicate what is observed, or to observe through expression – corresponding to what Henry James called "rendering" (2009/1904, p. xlvi). There is no means in principle or practice to distinguish between the acts of noting and the extraordinary artistry of literary expression demonstrated by the brothers. Yet that both of the brothers enjoyed and practiced what they considered to be observation, encouraging one another in noting and describing subtle variations in sensory qualities, is reflected in Henry's memoirs of their early lives together.

In several passages, Henry's remarks are reminiscent of the spirit of the earlier self-identified "observers":

"I ought to endeavor to keep, to a certain extent, a record of passing impressions, of all that comes, that goes, that I see, & feel, & observe.

To catch and keep something of life – that's what I mean." (Notebooks, p. 635; from *Henry James: Autobiographies*, Philip Horne, ed., 2016, Library of America)

"I speak as one who has had time to take many notes, to be struck with many differences, and to see, a little typically perhaps, what may eventually happen." (Other Autobiographical Writings, p. 714)

Important to note is that Henry's reference to being struck with differences seems strikingly similar to what stands out as the important ingredient in writing a careful case study, and converges with the sense of observation Hacking called the important one for experimental research – the "noticing" of difference in pattern. Of course the range of what is noticed is broader and more loosely defined when one is writing a novel (or case study, for that matter) in comparison with a focused experiment, but we are speaking here of the activity itself. The reference to seeing "a little typically" (a tentative generalizing from the observation of particulars), and even to a form of expectation (even "prediction") is also important to note in the passage provided. And the recording of noticed differences acknowledged by reference to taking notes speaks to the merger of noticing and expression in the act itself – that is, in practice.

The differences with which Henry James is "struck" invariably include the intricacies of the psychological realm and human relations. His published novels display an extraordinary level of observed detail in relation to characters and scenes, engaging the unarticulated experience of his characters in each of his published works and rendering the novels deeply psychological works, if not part of the formal literature of psychology. We could choose any single novel for example, but because of its reflection not only on the variabilities of personal experience but also on the interface of personal experiences with the social and political order (and disorder), we could do no better than *The Bostonians* (James, 2000/1886). A critic's review of *The Bostonians* shortly after it was published remarks upon characters "built up like a coral reef," and highlights the habits of thought James exhibits, equating "observation" with a "seizing upon" particular and characteristic features of the ways of life described:

> He comes back, as it were, to scenes once familiar to him, bringing with him habits of thought and observation which make him seize upon just those features of life which would arrest the attention of an Englishman or a Frenchman . . . he is caught by the queer variety of humanitarianism which with many people outside Boston is the peculiar attribute of that much suffering city. (Scudder, 1886)

In addition, Henry James builds into his descriptions of some characters a proclivity toward observation, a habit of seizing upon details as a way of being, but builds into his characterization differing styles or qualities of observational activity. In at least one case there is an implicit association with the scientific mind, in the depiction of Doctor Prance, a female physician who keeps a physiological laboratory in the basement. She is described with an "acute, suspicious eye" (p. 34), "tough and technical" (p. 34) as well as dedicated to science; "she pursued her medical studies far into the night" (p. 33). In his description, James seems to associate her "near-sighted deprecation" and distaste for generalization with her scientific interests:

> [S]he looked about her with a kind of near-sighted deprecation, and seemed to hope that she should not be expected to generalize in any way [sic], or supposed to have come up for any purpose more social than to see what Miss Birdseye wanted this time. (James, 2000/1886, p. 26)

In contrast, the character of Basil Ransom is inclined toward observation, but his observational habits are of the kind that catapult him to quick categorizations and generalizations, evident in his first reaction to Dr. Prance herself, wherein he is quick to generalize, to cast her as a perfect representative of a type, a type with whom he has little personal experience but impressions formed only from existing stereotypes, depicted as the "unregenerate imagination" of the south.

> Basil Ransom had already noticed Doctor Prance; he had not been at all bored, and had observed every one in the room, arriving at all sorts of ingenious inductions. The little medical lady struck him as a perfect example of the "Yankee female" – the figure which, in the unregenerate imagination of the children of the cotton-States, was produced by the New England school-system, the Puritan code, the ungenial climate, the absence of chivalry. (James, 2000/1886, p. 33)

Similarly, Dr. Prance's keen discernment of particulars is juxtaposed against the style of Verena Tarrant, whose inspired speaking impresses Basil Ransom as "full of school-girl phrases, of patches of remembered eloquence of childish lapses of logic, of flights of fancy which might indeed have had success at Topeka" (James, 2000/1886, p. 33). Scudder's review is not charitable in relation to James's portrayal of this character, asserting that she is "constructed for the purposes of the story, and is, we may say, a purely imaginary being." Similarly, of the Basil Ransom character, depicted as newly arrived from Mississippi: "we cannot resist the conviction that Mr. James has never been in Mississippi, as the phrase goes, and trusts to luck that his readers have not been there either"(Scudder, 1886).

Scudder's criticism of the artificial quality of some of *The Bostonians'* characters is in marked contrast to his praise of other characters, of which he says that one stands in amazement before the delicacy of workmanship. As an aside, the sense here conveyed is that there is a form of "truth" to the best character development in literary works, and however this "truth" is to be understood, it is accomplished through careful and fine-grained apprehension of distinguishing details – observation of actual persons, cultures, situations. When wrought successfully, the details facilitate abstraction, inference: "The astounding array of particulars invites one to pause and see if he cannot abstract the generals" (Scudder, 1886, Retrieved from https://www.theatlantic.com/past/docs/unbound/classrev/thebosto.htm).

In both his style as a writer and the traits he builds into his characters, Henry James displays an inclination toward "being observant" in the ordinary sense that Hacking regards as important to science. The importance of this discriminatory activity to the development of any taxonomy is so obvious as to need little elaboration beyond this point. What does require emphasis, however, is evidence of a similar style and a similar valuing of fine discrimination in the best writing of William James. He skillfully applies the noticing of differences to his meticulous description of variations in religious experiences, his case studies of concrete persons and situations he studies in order to characterize the important features of the varieties he names (James, 1987/1902). This is James as a qualitative psychologist, but we may find aspects of this same tendency in James's writings on general psychology in the *Principles* (2007/1890), the groundbreaking work of theory development that established his reputation as the founder of American psychology. A passage from his chapter on the emotions will serve to illustrate the careful phenomenological description he uses to distinguish "the subtler emotions," "cerebral forms of pleasure and displeasure," associated with "moral, intellectual, and aesthetic" experiences (p. 368) from "coarser" emotions associated, for example, with bodily threat, followed by the theoretical assertion that the secondary or subtle emotions are "grafted" upon "more primary" feeling (p. 469):

> A glow, a pang in the breast, a shudder, a fullness of the breathing, a flutter of the heart, a shiver down the back, a moistening of the eyes, a stirring in the hypogastrium, and a thousand unnamable symptoms

besides, may be felt the moment the beauty excites us. And these symptoms also result when we are excited by moral perceptions, as of pathos, magnanimity or courage. The voice breaks and the sob rises in the struggling chest, or the nostril dilates and the fingers tighten, whilst the heart beats, etc., etc. ... As a matter of fact, however, the moral and intellectual cognitions hardly ever do exist thus unaccompanied. (William James, 2007/1890, pp. 470–471)

The value of detail and careful observation in the "ordinary" sense we have discussed in this chapter is evident in the work of both James brothers despite differences in the aim and form of their work and in their personal styles of expression. Weinfurt (2003) characterizes James's style of scholarship as one that emphasizes the distinguishing approach James himself described as one variation or cognitive style in *The Sentiment of Rationality* (1879), specifically one that "seeks to become intimately familiar with the messy details that constitute experience" (Weinfurt, 2003, p. 407).

Imaginative Sense-Making: Metaphor

We need not venture far into the work of either James brother to recognize the importance of metaphor to the development and "rendering" of their central ideas.

William James advanced understandings of consciousness with the metaphors of stream, as well as fringe. Unlike Titchner's search for basic elements of mind, a project based on an analogy drawn from chemistry, James's metaphors are drawn from everyday life. David Leary credits James's early interest, even obsession, with drawing, especially landscape, as a factor in his artful depictions of consciousness:

Consciousness, then, does not appear to itself chopped up in bits. Such words as "chain" or "train" do not describe it fitly as it presents itself in the first instance. It is nothing jointed; it flows. A "river" or a "stream" are the metaphors by which it is most naturally described. In talking of it hereafter, let us call it the stream of thought, of consciousness, or of subjective life. (James, 2007/1890, p. 239)

We can see that James is self-consciously seeking the best metaphor for consciousness, and he rejects some possibilities that capture certain features, that of movement or connection, but do not adequately characterize the essential feature of its continuous flow. He also depicts consciousness as "a bird's life," in that "it seems to be made of an alteration of flights and perchings" (for analysis, see Araujo, 2017). Other examples (among many): "The sense of sameness is the very keel and backbone of our thinking" (p. 459).

"Feelings are the germ and starting point of cognition, thoughts the developed tree" (p. 222).

These examples help to illustrate how metaphors function for theoretical purposes, enabling the reader or listener to grasp by the configuration of the image constructed the essential features of the phenomenon described, or the relation between the corresponding aspects. The persuasive nature of naked-eye observation, so basic to our everyday functioning, is harnessed in metaphor; it is as compelling and convincing, yet what we are "seeing" are abstractions – consciousness, feeling, time perception, sense of sameness – things that have no material, sensible reality, but are "pictured" as features of everyday human activity and experience. The use of analogical models of this kind thus advances psychological theorizing and becomes a matter of method, not merely artifice.

David Leary's paper titled "William James and the Art of Understanding" summarizes what he calls "two major features in James's portrait of human understanding ... (a) that all knowledge, including science, is ultimately based on the finding of analogy, which is to say, on the finding of an appropriate, enlightening comparison or metaphor; and (b) that the analogies or metaphors in any field of knowledge, including science, are (or should be) always changing rather than fixed" (1992, p. 153). In William James we see the use of metaphor to advance psychological theorizing, especially in the *Principles* and *Briefer Course*, but as Leary notes, in his later work he also depicts philosophical concepts metaphorically. He is, of course, in the early work, a general psychologist, at a time when this meant "the Science of Mental Life, both of its phenomena and their conditions" (2007/1890, p. 1). The scope of psychology as a discipline at least in the United States had not yet reached the study of personality, mood, motivation, social relations, human development, organizational influence, or cultural conflict.

However, in Henry James's writings these topics are taken up with extraordinarily detailed description of the conscious life of his characters, in writing that is saturated with symbolic imagery and metaphor. In contrast to William James, Henry uses metaphor to express interpersonal struggles, frequently involving conflict, compromise, or dilemma. A compelling example is provided in his late period novel, *The Golden Bowl* (2009/1904), a novel that tackles the difficult subjects of marital discord and deceit, with the central motif of an antique bowl that appears perfect but is known to have a crack.

"Does one make a present," she asked, "of an object that contains to one's knowledge a flaw?"

"Well, if one knows of it one has only to mention it. The good faith," the man smiled, "is always there."

"And leave the person to whom one gives the thing, you mean, to discover it?"

"He wouldn't discover it – if you're speaking of a gentleman."

"I'm not speaking of any one in particular," Charlotte said.

"Well, whoever it might be. He might know – and he might try. But he wouldn't find."

She kept her eyes on him as if, though unsatisfied, mystified, she yet had a fancy for the bowl. "Not even if the thing should come to pieces?" And then as he was silent: "Not even if he should have to say to me 'The Golden Bowl is broken'?" (James, 2009/1904, pp. 86–87)

Yet through these narrative techniques, the novels and essays of Henry James develop a set of general and surprisingly contemporary themes that transcend the struggles of his characters and touch on human fault lines more generally: the tensions between personal fulfillment and family responsibilities, between autonomy and love, especially for women, and the troubling confrontation of old and new world values as these are enacted in cultural exchange. If these themes are not also the stuff of psychology in a broad sense, we must question whether we have limited our discipline to a place of questionable contemporary relevance.

Perspective-Taking

Henry James deliberately endeavored to take the perspective of persons whose life situation was vastly different from his own: a female child caught in the custody battle of divorcing parents in *What Maisie Knew* (2010/1897), a dying young woman in *The Wings of the Dove* (1902), for example. That his technique involved a kind of imaginative projection into the situation and consciousness of these characters is evident in his description of his process, a process that began in a vaguely formed image of such a character. Here, for example, he describes his interest in the dying woman and her experience, and the experience of those in relation to her: "The image so figured would be, at best, but half the matter; the rest would be all the picture of the struggle involved, the adventure brought about, the gain recorded or the loss incurred, the precious experience somehow compassed" (1934/1909, p. 288).

In his late period novels, Henry James experiments with a new narrative strategy, a new method, which abandons the usual technique of describing action and character experience from the point of view of a distanced, objective, omniscient story teller – "the impersonal author" (2009/1909, p. xli), and instead tells the story from the distinct points of view of two different characters. He refers to this technique as a system and a method, and in his preface to *The Golden Bowl* (2009/1909) attempts to describe his intent: "I nevertheless affect myself as having held my system fast and fondly, with one hand, at least, by the manner in which the whole thing remains subject to the register, ever so closely kept, of the consciousness of but two of the characters" (p. xlii). He explains why the register of the consciousness of these two in particular is vital to the narrative: [use block quote]"The Prince, in the first half of the book, virtually sees and knows and makes out, virtually represents to himself everything that concerns us – very nearly (though he doesn't speak in the first person) after the fashion of other reporters and critics of other situations. Having a consciousness highly susceptible of registration, he thus makes us see the things that may most interest us reflected in it as in the clean class held up to so many of the 'short stories' of our long list; and yet after all never a whit to the prejudice of his being just as consistently a foredoomed, entangled, embarrassed agent in the general imbroglio ... The function of the Princess [Maggie], in the remainder, matches exactly with his; the register of her consciousness is as closely kept" (pp. xlii–xliii). Therefore, as he summarizes the technique used, "With a like consistency we see the same persons and things again, but as Maggie's interest, her exhibitional charm, determines the view" (p. xliv).

The editor's introduction to *The Golden Bowl* notes James's refusal to speak from the superior view of "the omniscient narrator," and that it "was James's adoption of a partial view that enabled him to sidestep the spectacle of the Prince 'relating' to Charlotte ... what we see instead is the Prince feeling his way into a situation ... we see him through his own eyes" (p. xiii). The editor attributes the realness of the character to this literary technique.

During roughly the same time period, William James undertook his groundbreaking exploration of religious experience, and it is in this work that his own interest in and exploration of perspective-taking as a system or method is most on display. In *The Varieties of Religious Experience* (1987/1902), James exhibits awareness of all of the senses of perspective we noted in Chapter 5. He expresses his disciplinary identity explicitly, contrasts it with other disciplinary identities, and uses his own discipline to both defend his interest and guide the questions he feels entitled to address:

> I am neither a theologian, nor a scholar learned in the history of religion, nor an anthropologist. Psychology is the only branch of learning in which I am particularly versed. To the psychologist the religious propensities of man must be at least as interesting as any other of the facts pertaining to his mental constitution. It would seem, therefore, that as a psychologist, the natural thing for me would be to invite you to a descriptive survey of those religious propensities. (p. 12)

He also suggests that psychological inquiry is inherently a matter of perspective-taking, if what we mean by this includes an effort to understand the feelings and experiences of actual persons other than oneself: "If the inquiry be psychological, not religious institutions but religious feelings and religious impulses must be its subject." The most useful documents for such a pursuit will be from persons "best able to give an intelligible account of their ideas and motives" (1987/1902, p. 12).

James's goal of understanding and describing others' experience, which he closely aligns with the "empirical attitude," contrasts with the judgmental attitude persons exhibit in everyday interactions: "comments which unsentimental people so often pass on their more sentimental acquaintances" (p. 18), a "method of discrediting states of mind for which we have all antipathy," which we all use "to some degree in criticizing persons whose states of mind we regard as overstrained" (p. 19). It also contrasts with an academic stance in which the emphasis is on causal explanation of experiential states rather than understanding: "proclamations of the intellect bent on showing the existential conditions of absolutely everything," which lead to our feeling "menaced and negated in the springs of our innermost life" (1987/1902, p. 18).

Lacking religious feeling, religious experience in his own life, James is obliged to engage in something like perspective-taking in an effort to understand the experience of those persons who do have it. One of the most interesting examples of this effort is in his attempt to characterize the qualities of mystical experience:

> My constitution shuts me out from that enjoyment almost entirely, and I can speak of them only at second hand, but though forced to look upon the subject so externally, I will be as objective and receptive as I can; and I think I shall convince you of the reality of the states in question, and of the paramount importance of their function. (p. 342)

Through analysis of published narratives as well as interviews with acquaintances, James describes a "cosmic consciousness," the function of which he views "as distinct from any possessed by the average man as self-consciousness is distinct from any function possessed by one of the higher animals," for which he provides a taxonomy of the relevant aspects that appear to him characteristic of mystical states across religious traditions. Through James's investigation of religious experience we are also reminded of the difficulty of characterizing "perspective" as reducing to cultural or other group belonging. He does not distinguish "the Christian perspective" from "the Jewish perspective" from "the Buddhist perspective," but distinguishes mystical consciousness from the everyday, "healthy-minded" religious persons from those suffering under "the sick soul."

The Personal and Communal

It is difficult to clearly demarcate the aspects of the work of either James brother that fit cleanly into the category of art or science. Of particular interest is a remark Henry James makes that links the sensitive attunement to the particular features of situations, what he repeatedly calls "impressions" to the possibility of science: "Never did I quite shake it off, I think, that impressions might themselves be science – and this probably, because I didn't then know them, as anything but life . . . There was to come to me of course in time the due perception that neither was of the least use – use to myself – without the other" (*Notes of a Son and Brother*, 2016, p. 272). Both brothers employ (to full advantage) "observation" (i.e., the practice of noticing and describing details and relating the details to one another); they also use metaphor extensively and affirm the value of understanding a variety of perspectives. Without denying that the activity in question reflects normative structures and demands as these are negotiated in various levels of community (e.g., the scholarly context and community of each brother), their engagement in these activities is personal in the sense that their qualities, interests, style, and identities are intimately related to what is observed, reflected on, and thus passed along to others to evaluate. William described the relation of the activities of persons to what we might call the communal store of knowledge as a system in which we must participate to our best ability:

> Something is before us; we do our best to tell what it is, but in spite of our good will we may go astray, and give a description more applicable to some other sort of thing. The only safeguard is in the final consensus of our farther knowledge about the thing in question, later views correcting earlier ones, until at last the harmony of a consistent system is reached. Such a system, gradually worked out, is the best guarantee the

psychologist can give for the soundness of any particular psychologic observation which he may report. Such a system we ourselves must strive, as far as may be, to attain. (2007/1890, p. 192)

Henry expressed a similar idea in a passage on the responsibility of the artist and her relation to the social order:

The more we are capable of acting the less gropingly we plead such differences; whereby, with any capability, we recognize betimes that to "put" things is very exactly and responsibly and interminably to do them ... Our relation to them is essentially traceable, and in that fact abides, we feel, the incomparable luxury of the artist. It rests altogether with himself not to break with his values, not to "give away" his importances. Not to *be* disconnected, for the tradition of behavior, he has but to feel that he is no; by his lightest touch the whole chain of relation and responsibility is reconstituted. Thus if he is always doing he can scarce, by his own measure, ever have done. All of which means for him conduct with a vengeance, since it is conduct minutely and pub- lically [*sic*] attested. (2009/1909, p. lxi)

In light of the extraordinary powers of observation, imaginative sense- making, and perspective-taking the brothers separately and collectively exhibit, one might point to William and Henry James as exceptions rather than examples, attributing their achievements to rare brilliance and unique abilities. Clearly, one might note, Henry has "gifts," native talents that are different from those of his brother but that share a common foundation of noticing difference and similarity in situations, depicting them in colorful, evocative language, and affirming the value of occupying perspectives other than his own. Some people are better at these things; they have more facility and natural inclination. Yet we do the topic and our discipline a disservice by putting it down in its entirety to a matter of genetic endowment or gift. Attunement and attention and exploration of a variety of representational formats were things that were encouraged, modeled, *valued* in the family and by the associates of the family (e.g., see Menand, 2001). Importantly, too, we can find in a well-chosen case exam- ple vivid and obvious features that help us to understand and recognize similar cases. This is itself a literary point of art, a means of carrying meaning in general through a single and vivid example – the point of symbolic imagery in its varied forms, in its generalizing function, its representation of a world of relations beyond itself: "Unlike wanton designers, we had, not to create but simply to recognize – recognize that is, with the last fineness. The thing was to induce the vision of Portland

place to generalize itself . . . our business would be then to understand."
(James, 2009/1909, p. xlviii)

ART AND SCIENCE

Although the illustration through the James brothers may be a novel line of
comparison, one reflecting my own peculiar configuration of interest in
both science and the literary arts, I am hardly alone in noting deep
comparisons between artistic and scientific innovation, or in believing
that there is significance to these connections, and that they relate to
questions of values. As a recent example, Walter Isaacson's extraordinary
biography of Leonardo Da Vinci vividly illustrates the manifold ways his
subject's genius reflects his profound immersion in both artistic and
scientific/technological domains, and he notes that what made Leonardo
a genius was precisely "the ability to apply imagination to intellect."
To Isaacson, Leonardo's "facility for combining observation with fantasy
allowed him, like other creative geniuses, to make unexpected leaps that
related things seen to things unseen" (Isaacson, 2017, p. 518). Just as the
writings of the James brothers, Leonardo's supreme artistic achievement
provides a window into the connections between arts and sciences, and
Isaacson's facility in bringing these connections to the fore testifies to their
influence in his own formidable creative accomplishment, and to their
broader *value*.

Earlier, Bronowski argued for recognition of the "likeness between the
creative acts of the mind in art and in science" (1961, p. 6); "what the human
mind makes of the sense data, and thinks about, is always a created thing"
(p. 32). The similarity he noted is a reflection of the aesthetic value, of
passionate engagement and the *pleasure* inherent in creative movement in
both domains. He acknowledges that there are differences in the various
attitudes and goals, as well as in the fact that scientific models are formally
tested, refined, and revised according to their predictive accuracies.
Nevertheless, creative acts in the arts and sciences are distinguished primarily by the "degree of freedom" open to each, with scientists more
constrained by method, model, and the formal requirements imposed by
material. Qualitative studies of scientists repeatedly illustrate the interplay,
the synthesis of subjective and objective dimensions of scientific innovation (e.g., Osbeck & Nersessian, 2017; Wertheimer, 1981/1945). It is important to note that I am not suggesting that scientific reasoning in any
domain, psychology included, is a matter of subjectivity alone, only that
subjectivity – the personal – is an inescapable component of the mix.

Moreover, as Kuhn acknowledges, subjectivity includes not only emotions and identity, but personal reasoning and choice, the application of rationality but as influenced by learning history, including the problem-solving history that impacts convictions and stances taken in relation to theory selection and evaluation (Kuhn, 1977).

But although the personal aspect contributes to the forward movement of theory, it also points to reasons for caution, vigilance, and restraint. Scientists are human, with all of the frailty and variability that implies. An interesting essay by Kuhn written as a commentary to "Professor Hafner's rapprochement of science and art" acknowledges his general agreement with the thesis that there are "persistent parallels between the two enterprises I had been taught to regard as polar" (1977, p. 340), leading him to concur that "the more carefully we try to distinguish artist from scientist, the more difficult our task becomes" (p. 341). Yet for Kuhn this admission is "disquieting" rather than celebratory, and he purposefully seeks then highlights important differences between the enterprises of art and science that should not escape our gaze. The clearest contrast he finds is in the differences art and science exhibit in relation to their disciplinary past: "past products of artistic activity are still vital parts of the artistic scene"; in contrast, "science destroys its past" (p. 345). He also sees no response to internal crisis orienting change in the artistic community as it does in science and finds scientists unlikely to experiment with different "styles" of working in different periods of their lives. Such alteration on the part of the scientist would likely be judged as "wrong" rather than as a fresh approach to a subject matter as it would be for the artist.

Kuhn is speaking to a difference in norms as well as a difference in values between the communities he envisions. There are divergent identities in the communities of arts and sciences, with differing requirements for adaptation and successful performance within them, different standards by which the work is judged. The specific differences he sees may be contested; it is not self-evident that artists and scientists uniformly display radically different relations to their history. There are alternative possible theories of this relation, as well as variations in standards that might be observed between art forms, or between different scientific communities. That is, there are normative differences in any two academic communities, not only between disciplines but within disciplines, even within different laboratories in the same science. Regional differences also apply. In short, the question of the relation between arts and sciences, like the question of the continuity of science, is a matter for which there is good evidence on either side, and thus position taken is influenced by values, by those of the person taking this question as well as values reflective of broader cultural patterns and historical circumstance. It can hardly be accidental that Köhler and Malinowski separately offer strong statements of the interconnection of science and values during times of social turbulence and postwar devastation (in response to different wars).

Our own time seems similarly marred by challenge if not outright crisis in many directions and on many levels. In my view this is a time that calls for emphasis on points of similarity between arts and sciences for the reasons I have stressed repeatedly: to generate new resources for problem-solving, to facilitate interdisciplinary collaboration, and to imbue a needed sense of responsibility for the products of our making – psychological theories and practices. Both of these follow, similarly, from an emphasis on the person-hood of the researcher – the acting person of psychological science.

If in the example of the James brothers the analysis of the importance of acting persons seems too grounded in the nineteenth century, it is impor-tant to note that the emphasis bears on the possibility of cutting-edge or frontier theorizing against the extraordinarily complex challenges of our contemporary context. In philosophy of physics, Pandit and Dosch articu-late a central question for understanding the possibility of scientific pro-gress to better understand the kind of reasoning that makes frontier innovation possible: "The central question: What *kind of scientific reason-ing* is it within physics which triggers the dynamics of problem and theory development at its frontiers, keeping them open to scientific change?" The authors note the implications of this shift away from a body of knowledge as a collection of facts to a revisable resource for "fostering strategic interdisciplinary research at the newer and most challenging frontiers that have emerged in recent decades ... pushing humanity for more action for building interfaces between scientific disciplines caught in their separate past histories" (Pandit & Dosch, 2013, p. 300). I add only that the questions need to be broadened beyond interfaces between the sciences to the interfaces between the sciences and humanities, or science and the arts. It is only in these interfaces that the nature of psychological observa-tion and the full range of sense-making strategies available for tackling the new and challenging frontiers can be explored and understood.

FINAL THOUGHTS AND APPLICATIONS

We now consider what the implications of reimagined epistemic priorities might be, what they might mean for psychology as a discipline and voca-tion. At a minimum, an acting person framework for psychological science points to a need for open discussion and continuous evaluation of the criteria according to which psychology students are selected and the values that shape their education, enabling them to bring a wider range of talents and interests to bear on psychological questions, and, indeed, to broaden the range of questions defined as psychological. There is in general a need to prioritize qualities of thought over conformity to the rules of method, and a need to enhance engagement in the world of persons, the specific features of their particular situations, and to imagine what is possible in the direction of more just and sustainable conditions. There is also, as repeatedly noted, a need to join forces with other disciplines in the service of working creatively toward a better human future. There is little point in upholding old dichotomies and disciplinary boundaries unreflectively if they do not prove useful in addressing new demands.

Isaacson's study ends with a section titled "Learning from Leonardo" based on the premise that the life of the artist/inventor offers "a wealth of lessons" for contemporary readers (Isaacson, 2017, p. 519). The suggestions he makes are depicted as concrete activities, beginning with a suggestion to develop the habit of careful observation in everyday life. My purpose in depicting categories of activity as epistemic priorities was to imply that these activities are of value toward the project of addressing the challenges of a new frontier – the frontier of human challenge and the frontier of interdisciplinary collaboration needed to address it. If valued at the level of the psychological community, activities may be cultivated, encouraged, developed, pursued – in education, in training, and in the everyday habits of life.

REFERENCES

Adler, A. (1964). *The individual psychology of Alfred Adler.* H. L. Ansbacher & R. R. Ansbacher (eds.). New York: Harper Torchbooks.

Angell, J. R. (1904). *Psychology: An introductory study of the structure and function of human consciousness.* New York: Henry Holt.

Angell, J. R. (1907). The province of functional psychology. *Psychological Review,* 14, 61–91.

Angell, J. R. (1915). *Chapters from modern psychology.* New York: Longmans, Green, & Co.

Ansbacher, H. L., & Ansbacher, R. R. (eds.). (1956). *The individual psychology of Alfred Adler.* Oxford: Basic Books.

Araujo, S. F. (2016). *Wundt and the philosophical foundations of psychology.* London: Springer.

Araujo, S. F. (2017). Psychology between science and common sense: William James and the problems of psychological language in the Principles. *New Ideas in Psychology,* 46, 39–45.

Atkinson, P., & Hammersley, M. (1994). Ethnography and participant observation. In N. K. Denzin & Y. S. Lincoln (eds.), *Handbook of qualitative research* (pp. 248–261). Thousand Oaks: SAGE.

Austin, J. L. (1962). *How to do things with words.* Cambridge: Harvard University Press.

Baars, B. (1986). *The cognitive revolution in psychology.* New York: Guilford Press.

Bacon, F. (1937). In R. F. Jones (ed.), *Novum Organum.* New York: Odyssey Press, Inc., Originally published 1620.

Bacon, F. (1996). *Sylva Sylvarum: Or a natural history in ten centuries.* Whitefish, MT: Kessinger. Originally published posthumously 1627.

Baker, D. B., & Benjamin Jr., L. T. (2000). The affirmation of the scientist–practitioner: A look back at Boulder. *American Psychologist,* 55(2), 241–247.

Bender, A., & Beller, S. (2016). Current perspectives on cognitive diversity. *Frontiers in Psychology,* 7, 509. http://doi.org/10.3389/fpsyg.2016.00509

Bentley, M. (1929). "Observer" and "subject." *American Journal of Psychology,* 41, 682.

Bergner, R. M. (2017). What is a person? What is the self? Formulations for a science of psychology. *Journal of Theoretical and Philosophical Psychology*, 37 (2), 77–90.

Berlin, I., & Hardy, H. (1999). *The Roots of Romanticism: The AW Mellon Lectures in the Fine Arts 1965.* Washington, DC: The National Gallery of Art.

Black, M. (1955, June). XII.–Metaphor, *Proceedings of the Aristotelian Society*, Vol. 55, 1, pp. 273–294.

Black, M. (1962). *Models and metaphors: Studies in language and philosophy.* Ithaca: Cornell University Press.

Bloor, D. (1984). The strengths of the strong programme. In J. R. Brown (ed.), *Scientific rationality: The sociological turn* (pp. 75–94). Dordrecht: Reidel.

Bowlby, J. (1988). *A secure base: Clinical applications of attachment theory.* New York: Routledge.

Brentano, F. (1874). *Psychologie vom empirischen sandpunkte.* Leipzig: Duncker & Humblot.

Breuer, J., & Freud, S. (1957). *Studies on hysteria.* J. Strachey (ed.). Oxford: Basic Books, Inc. Originally published 1895, *Studien über Hysterie.*

Bridgman, P. (1959). *The way things are.* Cambridge: Harvard University Press.

Brightman, E. S. (1943). Personality as a metaphysical principle. In E. S. Brightman (ed.), *Personalism in theology* (pp. 40–63). Boston: Boston University Press.

Brockmeier, J. (2009). Reaching for meaning: Human agency and the narrative imagination. *Theory & Psychology*, 19(2), 213–233.

Bronowski, J. (1961). *Science and human values.* New York: Harper & Row. Originally published 1956.

Bruner, J. (1973. The conditions of creativity. In J. Bruner (ed.), *Beyond the information given* (pp. 208–217). New York: Norton & Co. Originally published 1962.

Bruner, J. (1973). Going beyond the information given. In J. Bruner (ed.), *Beyond the information given* (pp. 218–238). New York: Norton & Co. Originally published 1957.

Bruner, J. (1990). *Acts of meaning.* Cambridge: Harvard University Press.

Buford, T. (2006). Persons in the tradition of Boston Personalism. *The Journal of Speculative Philosophy*, 20(3), 214–218.

Burrow, R. (1999). *Personalism: A critical introduction.* St. Louis: Chalice Press.

Byford, J., & Tileagă, C. (2014). Social psychology, history, and the study of the Holocaust: The perils of interdisciplinary "borrowing". *Peace and Conflict: Journal of Peace Psychology*, 20(4), 349.

Camp, E. (2009). Two varieties of literary imagination: Metaphor, fiction, and thought experiments. *Midwest Studies in Philosophy*, 33(1), 107–130.

Cartwright, N. (1997). Models: The blueprints for laws. *Philosophy of Science*, 64, S292–S303.

Chalmers, A. (1999). *What is this thing called science?* 3rd ed. Indianapolis: Hackett. Originally published 1976.

Chalmers, A. (2013). *What is this thing called science?* 4th ed. Indianapolis: Hackett. Originally published 1976.

Ciarrochi, J., Morin, A. J. S., Sahdra, B. K., Litalien, D., & Parker, P. D. (2017). A longitudinal person-centered perspective on youth social support: Relations with psychological wellbeing. *Developmental Psychology*, 53(6), 1154–1169.

Cokely, E. T., & Feltz, A. (2014). Expert intuition. In L. Osbeck & B. Held (eds.), *Rational intuition* (pp. 213–238). New York: Cambridge University Press.

Comte, A. (1957). *A general view of positivism.* J. H. Bridges, trans. New York: Speller. Original work published 1849.

Coplan, A., & Goldie, P. (eds.). (2011). *Empathy: Philosophical and psychological perspectives.* Oxford: Oxford University Press.

Crenshaw, K. (1989). Demarginalizing the intersection of race and sex: A black feminist critique of antidiscrimination doctrine, feminist theory, and anti-racist politics. *University of Chicago Legal Forum:* special issue, *Feminism in the Law: Theory, Practice, and Criticism*, University of Chicago Law School, 139–168.

Cronbach, L. J. (1957). The two disciplines of scientific psychology. *American Psychologist*, 12(11), 671–684.

Danziger, K. (1990). *Constructing the subject: Historical origins of psychological research.* Cambridge: Cambridge University Press.

Danziger, K. (1997). *Naming the mind.* London: SAGE.

Danziger, K. (2013). Historical psychology of persons: Categories and practice. In J. Martin & M. Bickhard (eds.), *The psychology of personhood: Philosophical, historical, social-developmental, and narrative perspectives* (pp. 51–80). New York: Cambridge University Press.

Dashiell, J. F. (1929). Note on use of term "observer." *Psychological Review*, 36, 550–551.

Daston, L. (1998). Fear and loathing of the imagination in science. *Daedalus*, 127(1), 73–95.

Daston, L. (2011). The empire of observation. In L. Daston & E. Lunbeck (eds.), *Histories of scientific observation* (pp. 81–114). Chicago: University of Chicago Press.

Date, G., & Chandrasekharan, S. (2017): Beyond efficiency: Engineering for sustainability requires solving for pattern. *Engineering Studies.* https://doi.org/10.1080/19378629.2017.1410160

De Jaegher, H., & Di Paolo, E. (2007). Participatory sense-making: An enactive approach to social cognition. *Phenomenology and the Cognitive Sciences*, 6, 485–507.

Derry, S., & Schunn, C. (2014). Interdisciplinarity: A beautiful but dangerous beast. In S. Derry, C. Schunn, & M. Gernsbacher (eds.), *Interdisciplinary collaboration: An emerging cognitive science* (pp. xiii–xx). New York: Psychology Press.

Derry, S., Schunn, C., & Gernsbacher, M. (eds.). (2014). *Interdisciplinary collaboration: An emerging cognitive science.* New York: Psychology Press.

Dewey, J. (1910). *How we think.* New York: Heath.

Dewey, J. (1938). *Logic: The theory of inquiry.* New York: Holt, Rinehart & Winston.

Dewey, J. (2008). Experience and nature. In J. A. Boydston (ed.), *The later works of John Dewey*, Vol. 1. Carbondale: Southern Illinois University Press.

Dewey, J., & Bentley, A. (1949). The knower and the known. *The Later Works of John Dewey*, 16. Boston: Beacon.

Dilthey, W. (1977). Ideas concerning a descriptive and analytic psychology. In R. Zaner & K. Heiges (trans.), *Descriptive psychology and historical understanding* (pp. 21–120). Dordrecht: Springer. Originally published 1894.

Donoghue, D. (2014). *Metaphor.* Cambridge: Harvard University Press.

Douglas, H. (2009). *Science, policy, and the value-free ideal.* Pittsburgh: University of Pittsburgh Press.

Dupré, J. (1993). *The disorder of things.* Cambridge: Harvard University Press.

Elgin, C. Z. (2014). Fiction as thought experiment. *Perspectives on Science,* 22(2), 221–241.

Elliott, K. C. (2017). *A tapestry of values: An introduction to values in science.* New York: Oxford University Press.

Elms, A. C. (1975). The crisis of confidence in social psychology. *American Psychologist,* 30(10), 967–976.

Emerson, R. M., Fretz, R. I., & Shaw, L. L. (2001). Participant observation and fieldnotes. In P. Atkinson, A. Coffey, S. Delamont, J. Lofland, & L. Lofland (eds.), *Handbook of ethnography* (pp. 352–368). London: SAGE Publications.

Emirbayer, M., & Goldberg, C. A. (2005). Pragmatism, Bourdieu, and collective emotions in contentious politics. *Theory and Society,* 34(5), 469–518.

Erikson, E. H. (1968). *Identity.* New York: Norton.

Feist, G. J. (2008). *The psychology of science and the origins of the scientific mind.* New Haven: Yale University Press.

Feyerabend, P. (1975). *Against method.* Scranton: Verso.

Fisher, H. (2017) Person, psychologist, and psychology suspended in a phase 1 science. *Theory & Psychology,* 27(4), 524–549.

Flanagan, O. J. (1981). Psychology, progress, and the problem of reflexivity: A study in the epistemological foundations of psychology. *Journal of the History of the Behavioral Sciences,* 17(3), 375–386.

Fox Keller, E. (1995). *Reflections on gender and science.* New Haven: Yale University Press.

Frappier, M., Meynell, L., & Brown, J. R. (eds.). (2012). *Thought experiments in philosophy, science, and the arts* (Vol. 11). Abingdon and New York: Routledge.

Freeman, M. (2014). *The priority of the other: Thinking and living beyond the self.* Oxford: Oxford University Press.

Frigg, R., & Hunter, M. (eds.). (2010). *Beyond mimesis and convention: Representation in art and science* (Vol. 262). New York: Springer Science & Business Media.

Gendler, T. S. (2004). Thought experiments rethought – and reperceived. *Philosophy of Science,* 71, 1152–1163.

Gentner, D. (1983). Structure-mapping: A theoretical framework for analogy. *Cognitive Science,* 7(2), 155–170.

Gergen, K. J. (1973). Social psychology as history. *Journal of Personality and Social Psychology,* 26(2), 309–320.

Gergen, K. J. (1985). The social constructionist movement in modern psychology. *American Psychologist,* 40(3), 266–275.

Gergen, K. J. (1990). Metaphor, metatheory, and the social world. In D. Leary (ed.), *Metaphor in the history of psychology* (pp. 267–299). New York: Cambridge University Press.

Gergen, K. J. (2001). Preface. In K. Gergen (ed.), *Social construction in context* (pp. ix–x). London: SAGE.

Gesn, P. R., & Ickes, W. (1999). The development of meaning contexts for empathic accuracy: Channel and sequence effects. *Journal of Personality and Social Psychology*, 77(4), 746–761.

Giere, R. N. (1999). Using models to represent reality. In L. Magnani, N. Nersessian, & P. Thagard (eds.), *Model-based reasoning in scientific discovery* (pp. 41–57). New York: Kluwer.

Giere, R. N. (2010). *Scientific perspectivism*. Chicago: University of Chicago Press.

Giorgi, A. (1970). *Psychology as a human science: A phenomenologically based approach*. Oxford: Harper & Row.

Goertzen, J. R. (2008). On the possibility of unification: The reality and nature of the crisis in psychology. *Theory & Psychology*, 18(6), 829–852.

Gooding, D. (1990). *Experiment and the making of meaning*. Dordrecht: Kluwer.

Gorman, S., & Gorman, J. (2017). *Denying to the grave: Why we ignore the facts that will save us*. New York: Oxford University Press.

Gould, S. (ed.). (2001). *The value of science: Essential writings of Henri Poincaré*. New York: Modern Library.

Greenwood, J. D. (2015). *A conceptual history of psychology: Exploring the tangled web*. Cambridge: Cambridge University Press.

Grice, J., Barrett, P., Cota, L., Felix, C., Taylor, Z., Garner, S., & Vest, A. (2017). Four bad habits of modern psychologists. *Behavioral Sciences*, 7(3), 53.

Gruber, H. (1974). *Darwin on man: A psychological study of scientific creativity*. New York: Dutton.

Guba, E. G. (ed.). (1990a). *The paradigm dialog*. Thousand Oaks: SAGE.

Guba, E. G. (1990b). The alternative paradigm dialog. In E. G. Guba (ed.), *The paradigm dialog* (pp. 17–30). Thousand Oaks: SAGE.

Hacking, I. (1983). *Representing and intervening: Introductory topics in the philosophy of natural science*. New York: Cambridge University Press.

Hadamard, J. (1945). *The mathematician's mind: The psychology of invention in the mathematical field*. Princeton: Princeton University Press.

Haig, B. D. (2014). *Investigating the psychological world: Scientific method in the behavioral sciences*. Cambridge: MIT Press.

Hanson, N. R. (1958). *Patterns of discovery*. Cambridge: Cambridge University Press.

Haraway, D. (1988). Situated knowledges: The science question in feminism and the privilege of partial perspective. *Feminist Studies*, 14(3), 575–599.

Harding, S. G. (1986). *The science question in feminism*. Ithaca: Cornell University Press.

Harding, S. G. (2015). *Objectivity and diversity: Another logic of scientific research*. Chicago: University of Chicago Press.

Harré, R. (1992). What is real in psychology: A plea for persons. *Theory & Psychology*, 2(2), 153–158.

Harré, R. (2012). Positioning theory: Moral dimensions of social-cultural psychology. In J. Valsiner (ed.), *The Oxford handbook of culture and psychology* (pp. 196–206). Oxford: Oxford University Press.

Harré, R., & Krausz, M. (1995). *Varieties of relativism*. Oxford: Blackwell.

Hartley, D. (2013). *Observations on man: His frame, his duty, and his expectations.* Cambridge: Cambridge University Press. Originally published 1749.

Heidbreder, E. (1933). *Seven psychologies.* Englewood Cliffs: Prentice-Hall.

Henriques, G. (2003). The tree of knowledge system and the theoretical unification of psychology. *Review of General Psychology,* 7(2), 150–182.

Hesse, M. (1963). *Models and analogies in science.* London: Sheed and Ward.

Higgins, A. (1991).The just community approach to moral education: Evolution of the idea and recent findings. In W. M. Kurtines & J. L. Gewirtz (eds.), *Handbook of moral behavior and development,* Vol.3 (pp. 111–141). Hillsdale: Erlbaum.

Hockney, D. (1975). The bifurcation of scientific theories and indeterminacy of translation. *Philosophy of Science,* 42(4), 411–427.

Hoffman, M. L. (2001). *Empathy and moral development: Implications for caring and justice.* Cambridge: Cambridge University Press.

Hoffman, R. (1980). Metaphor in science. In R. P. Honeck & R. R. Hoffman (eds.), *Cognitive psychology and figurative language.* Hillsdale: L. Erlbaum.

Hoffman, E., Myerberg, N. R., & Morawski, J. G. (2015). Acting otherwise: Resistance, agency, and subjectivities in Milgram's studies of obedience. *Theory & Psychology,* 25(5), 670–689.

Hofstadter, D. (1995). A review of *Mental Leaps: Analogy in Creative Thought. AI Magazine,* 16(3), 75.

Hofstadter, D., & Sander, E. (2013). *Surfaces and essences: Analogy as the fuel and fire of thinking.* New York: Basic Books.

Hudson, R. 2014. *Seeing things: The philosophy of reliable observation.* New York: Oxford University Press.

Hutto, D. D., & Myin, E. (2017). *Evolving enactivism: Basic minds meet content.* Cambridge: MIT Press.

Isaacson, W. (2017). *Leonardo Da Vinci.* New York: Simon & Schuster.

James, H. (1934). *The art of the novel.* New York: Charles Scribner & Sons. Originally published 1909.

James, H. (2000). *The Bostonians.* London: Penguin Books. Originally published 1886, Macmillan & Co.

James, H. (2009). *The golden bowl.* Oxford: Oxford University Press. Originally published 1904; author's preface published 1909.

James, H. (2010). *What Maisie knew.* London: Penguin Classics. Originally published 1897.

James, H. (2016). A small boy and others. In P. Horne (ed.), *Henry James: Autobiographies* (pp. 1–250). New York: Library of America.

James, W. (1878). Remarks on Spencer's definition of mind as correspondence. *Journal of Speculative Philosophy,* XII (1), 1–18.

James, W. (1879). The sentiment of rationality. *Mind,* 4(15), 317–346.

James, W. (1890). *The principles of psychology,* Vols. 1 & 2. New York: Henry Holt.

James, W. (1892). *Psychology, the briefer course.* New York: Henry Holt.

James, W. (1987). *The varieties of religious experience: A study in human nature. Being the Gifford Lectures on Natural Religion Delivered at Edinburgh in 1901–1902.* In William James, *Writings 1902–1910,* pp. 1–478. New York: Library of America. Originally published 1902.

James, W. (2003). *Pragmatism: A new name for some old ways of thinking.* B. Vescio (ed.). New York: Barnes & Noble. Originally published 1907.

James, W. (2007). *The principles of psychology,* Vol. 1. New York: Cosimo Classics. Originally published 1890.

Johnson, M. (2007). *The meaning of the body.* Chicago: University of Chicago Press.

Johnson-Laird, P. N. (1983). *Mental models: Towards a cognitive science of language, inference, and consciousness (No. 6).* Boston: Harvard University Press.

Josselson, R., & Hopkins, B. (2015). Narrative psychology and life stories. In J. Martin, J. Sugarman, & K. Slaney (eds.), *The Wiley handbook of theoretical and philosophical psychology* (pp. 219–233). New York: Wiley.

Kant, I. (1960). *Observations on the feeling of the beautiful and sublime.* J. Goldthwait (trans.). Berkeley: University of California Press. Originally published 1764.

Kellert, S. H., Longino, H. E., & Waters, C. K. (eds.). (2006). *Scientific pluralism [electronic resource] (Vol. 19).* Minneapolis: University of Minnesota Press.

Kelly, G. A. (1955). *The psychology of personal constructs. Volume 1: A theory of personality.* New York: W.W. Norton.

Kim, U. (1990). Indigenous psychology: Science and applications. In R. W. Brislin (ed.), *Cross-cultural research and methodology series, Vol. 14. Applied cross-cultural psychology* (pp. 142–160). Thousand Oaks: Sage Publications, Inc.

Kind, A. (ed.). (2016). *The Routledge handbook of philosophy of imagination.* Abingdon and New York: Routledge.

Kirschner, S. R. (2006). Psychology and pluralism: Toward the psychological studies. *Journal of Theoretical and Philosophical Psychology,* 26(1–2), 1–17.

Kitcher, P. (1993). *The advancement of science: Science without legend, objectivity without illusions.* New York: Oxford University Press.

Kitcher, P. (2001). *Science, truth, and democracy.* New York: Oxford University Press.

Knorr-Cetina, K. D. (2013). *The manufacture of knowledge: An essay on the constructivist and contextual nature of science.* Oxford: Elsevier.

Koch, S. (1981). The nature and limits of psychological knowledge: Lessons of a century qua "science." *American Psychologist,* 36(3), 257–269.

Koch, S. (1993). "Psychology" or "the psychological studies"? *American Psychologist,* 48(8), 902–904.

Köhler, W. (1938). *The place of value in a world of facts.* Oxford: Liveright.

Köhler, W. (1973). *The mentality of apes.* London: Routledge & Kegan Paul. Originally published 1925.

Kounios, J., & Beeman, M. (2015). *The eureka factor: Aha moments, creative insight, and the brain.* New York: Random House.

Kraus, M. (2017). Voice-only communication enhances empathic accuracy. *American Psychologist,* 72(7), 644–654.

Kuhn, T. (1962). *Structure of scientific revolutions.* Chicago: University of Chicago Press.

Kuhn, T. (1977). *The essential tension.* Chicago: University of Chicago Press.

Lacey, H. (1999a). *Is science value free? Values and scientific understanding.* London: Routledge.

Lacey, H. (1999b). On cognitive and social values: A reply to my critics. *Science & Education*, 8(1), 89–103.

Lakoff, G., & Johnson, M. (2003). *Metaphors we live by*. Chicago: University of Chicago Press.

Lamiell, J. T. (2009). Reviving person-centered inquiry in psychology: Why it's erstwhile dormancy? In J. Valsiner, P. C. M. Molenaar, M. C. D. P. Lyra, & N. Chaudhary (eds.), *Dynamic process methodology in the social and developmental sciences* (pp. 31–44). New York: Springer.

Latour, B., & Woolgar, S. (1979). *Laboratory life: The construction of scientific facts*. Princeton: Princeton University Press.

Lauden, L. (1984). *Science and values*. Berkeley: University of California Press.

Leary, D. E. (1990). Psyche's muse: The role of metaphor in the history of psychology. In D. E. Leary (ed.), *Metaphors in the history of psychology* (pp. 1–78). New York: Cambridge University Press.

Leary, D. E. (1992). William James and the art of human understanding. *American Psychologist*, 47(2), 152–160.

Leonelli, S. (2016). *Data-centric biology: A philosophical study*. Chicago: University of Chicago Press.

Levitt, H. M., Motulsky, S. L., Wertz, F. J., Morrow, S. L., & Ponterotto, J. G. (2017). Recommendations for designing and reviewing qualitative research in psychology: Promoting methodological integrity. *Qualitative Psychology*, 4(1), 2–22.

Lewin, K. (1946). Behavior and development as a function of the total situation. Reprinted in D. Cartwright (ed.), *Field theory in social science: Selected papers by Kurt Lewin* (pp. 238–303). New York: Harper Torch Books, 1951.

Lincoln, Y. S. (1990). The making of a constructivist: A remembrance of transformations past. In E. Guba (ed.), *The paradigm dialog* (pp. 46–66). Newbury Park: Sage.

Lincoln, Y. S., & Guba, E. G. (1985). *Naturalistic inquiry* (Vol. 75). Beverly Hills: Sage.

Longino, H. (1983). Beyond "bad science": Skeptical reflections on the value-freedom of scientific inquiry. *Science, Technology, & Human Values*, 8 (1), 7–17.

Longino, H. (1990). *Science as social knowledge: Value and objectivity in scientific inquiry*. Princeton: Princeton University Press.

Longino, H. E. (1996). Cognitive and non-cognitive values in science: Rethinking the dichotomy. In L. Hankinson & J. Nelson (eds.), *Feminism, science, and the philosophy of science* (pp. 39–58). Dordrecht: Springer.

Longino, H. E. (2002). *The fate of knowledge*. Princeton: Princeton University Press.

Longino, H. E. (2004). How values can be good for science. In P. K. Machamer & G. Wolters (eds.), *Science, values, and objectivity* (pp. 127–142). Pittsburgh: University of Pittsburgh Press.

Mach, E. (1976). *Knowledge and error: Sketches on the psychology of enquiry*. T. J. McCormack & P. Filches, trans. Dordrecht: D. Reidel. Original work published 1905.

Machamer, P., & Osbeck, L. (2004). The social in the epistemic. In P. Machamer & G. Wolters (eds.), *Science, values, and objectivity* (pp. 1–13). Pittsburgh: University of Pittsburgh Press.

Machamer, P., & Wolters, G. (2004). Introduction. In P. Machamer & G. Wolters (eds.), *Science, values, and objectivity* (pp. 78–89). Pittsburgh: University of Pittsburgh Press.

MacLeod, M., & Nersessian, N. J. (2015). Modeling systems-level dynamics: Understanding without mechanistic explanation in integrative systems biology. *Studies in History and Philosophy of Science Part C: Studies in History and Philosophy of Biological and Biomedical Sciences*, 49, 1–11.

Magnani, L., Nersessian, N., & Thagard, P. (eds.). (1999). *Model-based reasoning in scientific discovery*. Dordrecht: Kluwer.

Mahoney, M. (2004). *Scientist as subject: The psychological imperative*. Cambridge: Ballinger. Originally published 1976.

Malone, K., & Barbarino, G. (2009). Narrations of race in STEM settings: Identity formation and its discontents. *Science Education*, 93(3), 485–510.

Martin, J. (2017). Studying persons in context: Taking social psychological reality seriously. *New Ideas in Psychology*, 44: 28–33.

Martin, J., & Bickhard, M. (2013). Introducing persons and the psychology of personhood. In J. Martin & M. Bickhard (eds.), *The psychology of personhood: Philosophical, historical, social-developmental, and narrative perspectives* (pp. 1–17). New York: Cambridge University Press.

Martin, J., Sugarman, J., & Hickenbottom, S. (eds.). (2010). *Persons: Understanding psychological selfhood and agency*. New York: Springer.

Masterman, M. (1970). The nature of a paradigm. In I. Lakatos & A. Musgrave (eds.), *Criticism and the growth of knowledge* (pp. 59–89). London: Cambridge University Press.

Matravers, D. (2010). Why we should give up on the imagination. *Midwest Studies in Philosophy*, 34(1), 190–199.

Maxwell, S. E., Lau, M. Y., & Howard, G. S. (2015). Is psychology suffering from a replication crisis? What does "failure to replicate" really mean? *American Psychologist*, 70(6), 487–498.

McAdams, D. P. (2014). The life narrative at midlife. *New Directions for Child and Adolescent Development*, 2014 (145), 57–69.

McAllister, J. (2012). Thought experiment and the exercise of imagination in science. In M. Frappier, L. Meynell, & J. R. Brown (eds.), *Thought experiments in philosophy, science, and the arts* (pp. 11–29). New York: Routledge.

McDaniel, K. (2014). Edith Stein: On the problem of empathy. In E. Schliesser (ed.), *Ten neglected philosophical classics*. Oxford: Oxford University Press.

Mead, G. H. (1934). *Mind, self and society* (Vol. 111). Chicago: University of Chicago Press.

Meltzoff, A. N. (2002). Imitation as a mechanism of social cognition: Origins of empathy, theory of mind, and the representation of action. In U. Goswami (ed.), *Blackwell handbook of childhood cognitive development* (pp. 6–25). Oxford: Blackwell.

Menand, L. (2001). *The metaphysical club: A story of ideas in America*. New York: Farrar, Straus and Giroux.

Menary, R. (2007). *Cognitive integration: Mind and cognition unbounded*. New York: Palgrave Macmillan.

Mill, J. S. (1882). *August Comte and positivism*, 3rd ed. London: Trübner.

Miller, R. B. (2004). *Facing human suffering: Psychology and psychotherapy as moral engagement.* Washington, D.C.: American Psychological Association.

Mills, J. A. (2010). Incorporating realist fiction into dialogical theories of the self. *Theory & Psychology, 20*(5), 621–640.

Mitchell, S. D. (2002). Integrative pluralism. *Biology and Philosophy, 17*(1), 55–70.

Mitroff, I. (1974). *The subjective side of science: Philosophical inquiry into the psychology of the Apollo Moon Scientists.* Amsterdam: Elsevier.

Moghaddam, F.M. (2004). From "psychology in literature" to "psychology is literature." *Theory & Psychology, 14*(4), 505–525.

Morawski, J. G. (1988). *The rise of experimentation in American psychology.* New Haven: Yale University Press.

Morawski, J. G. (2005). Reflexivity and the psychologist. *History of the Human Sciences, 18*(4), 77–105.

Morrow, S. L. (2005). Quality and trustworthiness in qualitative research in counseling psychology. *Journal of Counseling Psychology, 52*(2), 250–260.

Moser, K. S. (2000). Metaphor analysis in psychology – Method, theory, and fields of application. In *Forum Qualitative Sozialforschung/Forum: Qualitative Social Research, 1*(2), Art 21.

Muelder, W. G. (1998). Foreword. In R. Burrow, *Personalism: A critical introduction* (pp. x–xiii). St. Louis: Chalice Press.

Nemetz, A. (1958). Metaphor: The Daedalus of discourse. *Thought, 33*(3), 417–442.

Nersessian, N. (1984). *Faraday to Einstein: Constructing meaning in scientific theories.* Dordrecht: Martinus Nijhoff/Kluwer.

Nersessian, N. J. (1992). How do scientists think? Capturing the dynamics of conceptual change in science. *Cognitive Models of Science, 15*, 3–44.

Nersessian, N. J. (1999). Model-based reasoning in conceptual change. In L. Magnani, N. Nersessian, & P. Thagard (eds.), *Model-based reasoning in scientific discovery* (pp. 5–22). New York: Kluwer.

Nersessian, N. J. (2002). The cognitive basis of model-based reasoning in science. In P. Carruthers, S. Stitch, & M. Siegal (eds.), *The cognitive basis of science* (pp. 133–153). Cambridge: Cambridge University Press.

Nersessian, N. (2005). Interpreting scientific and engineering practices: Integrating the cognitive, social, and cultural dimensions. In M. E. Gorman, R. D. Tweney, D. C. Gooding, & A. P. Kincannon (eds.), *Scientific and technological thinking* (pp. 17–56). Hillsdale: Erlbaum.

Nersessian, N. J. (2008). *Creating scientific concepts.* Cambridge: MIT Press.

Nersessian, N. J. (2012). Engineering concepts: The interplay between concept formation and modeling practices in bioengineering sciences. *Mind, Culture, and Activity, 19*(3), 222–239.

Ortner, S. (1995). Resistance and the problem of ethnographic refusal. *Comparative Studies in Society and History, 37*(1), 173–193.

Osbeck, L. M. (1993). Social constructionism and the pragmatic standard. *Theory & Psychology, 3*(3), 337–349.

Osbeck, L. M. (1995). Social constructionism and the pragmatic standard revisited: A reply to Botschner. *Theory & Psychology, 5*(1), 153–157.

Osbeck, L. M. (2005). Method and theoretical psychology. *Theory & Psychology, 15*(1), 5–26.

Osbeck, L. M., & Held, B. S. (eds.). (2014). *Rational intuition: Philosophical roots, scientific investigations.* New York: Cambridge University Press.

Osbeck, L. M., & Nersessian, N. J. (2006). The Distribution of Representation. *Journal for the Theory of Social Behaviour,* 36(2), 141–160.

Osbeck, L. M., & Nersessian, N. J. (2010). Forms of positioning in interdisciplinary science practice and their epistemic effects. *Journal for the Theory of Social Behaviour,* 40(2), 136–161.

Osbeck, L. M., & Nersessian, N. J. (2012). The acting person in scientific practice. In R. Proctor & J. Capaldi (eds.), *Psychology of science: Implicit and explicit reasoning* (pp. 89–111). New York: Oxford University Press.

Osbeck, L. M., & Nersessian, N. J. (2013). Beyond motivation and metaphor: "Scientific passions" and anthropomorphism. In *EPSA11 Perspectives and Foundational Problems in Philosophy of Science* (pp. 455–466). Cham: Springer International.

Osbeck, L. M., & Nersessian, N. J. (2015). Prolegomena to an empirical philosophy of science. In S. Wagenknecht, N. J. Nersessian, & H. Andersen (eds.), *Empirical philosophy of science: Introducing qualitative methods into philosophy of science* (pp. 13–35). Cham: Springer International.

Osbeck, L. M., & Nersessian, N. J. (2017). Epistemic identities in interdisciplinary science. *Perspectives on Science,* 25(2), 226–260.

Osbeck, L. M., Nersessian, N. J., Malone, K. R., & Newstetter, W. C. (2011). *Science as psychology: Sense-making and identity in science practice.* Cambridge: Cambridge University Press.

Pandit, G. L., & Dosch, H. G. (2013). *The frontiers of theory development in physics: A methodological study in its dynamical complexity.* Los Angeles: Trebol Press.

Park, K. (2011). Observation in the margins, 500–1500. In L. Daston & E. Lunbeck (eds.), *Histories of scientific observation* (pp. 15–44). Chicago: University of Chicago Press.

Parker, I. (2015). *Critical discursive psychology,* 2nd ed. London: Palgrave Macmillan.

Peirce, C. S. (1868). Questions concerning certain faculties claimed for man. *The Journal of Speculative Philosophy,* 2(2), 103–114.

Piaget, J. (1962). *Play, dreams and imitation in children.* New York: Norton.

Plotkin, H. C. (2002). *The imagined world made real: Towards a natural science of culture.* New Brunswick: Rutgers University Press.

Poincaré, H. (2001a). The value of science. In S. J. Gould (ed.), *The value of science: Essential writings of Henri Poincaré* (pp. 181–337). New York: Modern Library. Originally published 1913.

Poincaré, H. (2001b). Science and method. In S. J. Gould (ed.), *The value of science: Essential writings of Henri Poincaré* (pp. 357–558). New York: Modern Library. Originally published 1914.

Polanyi, M. (1964). *Science, faith, and society.* Chicago: University of Chicago Press. Originally published 1946.

Polanyi, M. (1974). *Personal knowledge: Towards a post-critical philosophy.* Chicago: University of Chicago Press. Originally published 1958.

Polya, G. (1945). *How to solve it.* Princeton: Princeton University Press.

Pomata, G. (2011). Observation rising: Birth of an epistemic genre, 1500–1650. In L. Daston & E. Lunbeck (eds.), *Histories of scientific observation* (pp. 45–80). Chicago: University of Chicago Press.

Ponterotto, Joseph G. (2005). Qualitative research in counseling psychology: A primer on research paradigms and philosophy of science. *Journal of Counseling Psychology, 52*(2), 126–136.

Power, C., Higgins, A., & Kohlberg, L. (1989). *Lawrence Kohlberg's approach to moral education: A study of three democratic high schools.* New York: Columbia University Press.

Pribram, K. H. (1990). From metaphors to models: The use of analogy in neuropsychology. In David E. Leary (ed.), *Metaphors in the history of psychology* (pp. 79–103). Cambridge: Cambridge University Press.

Price, D. D., & Barrell, J. J. (2012). *Inner experience and neuroscience: Merging both perspectives.* Cambridge: MIT Press.

Proctor, R. (1991). *Value-free science? Purity and power in modern knowledge.* Cambridge: Harvard University Press.

Proctor, R. W., & Capaldi, E. J. (2006). *Why science matters: Understanding the methods of psychological research.* Malden: Blackwell.

Putnam, H. (1981). *Reason, truth and history.* Cambridge: Cambridge University Press.

Rabinow, P., & Bennett, G. (2012). *Designing human practices: An experiment with synthetic biology.* Chicago: University of Chicago Press.

Rabinow, P., & Stavrianakis, A. (2013). *Demands of the day: On the logic of anthropological inquiry.* Chicago: University of Chicago Press.

Robinson, D. N. (2014). Science, scientism, and explanation. In D. Williams & D. N. Robinson, *Scientism: The new orthodoxy* (pp. 23–40). London: Bloomsbury.

Rogers, C. R. (1963). Toward a science of the person. *Journal of Humanistic Psychology, 3*(2), 72–92.

Ross, W. D. (1928). *Complete works of Aristotle.* Oxford: Clarendon Press.

Sarbin, T. R. (1986). *Narrative psychology: The storied nature of human conduct.* Westport: Praeger/Greenwood.

Sarbin, T. R. (1993). The narrative as the root metaphor for contextualism. In S. C. Hayes, L. J. Hayes, H. W. Reese, & T. R. Sarbin (eds.), *Varieties of scientific contextualism* (pp. 51–65). Reno: Context Press.

Schatzman, L., & Strauss, A. (1973). *Field research: Strategies for a natural sociology.* London: Pearson.

Schön, D. (1963). *Displacement of concepts.* London: Tavistock Publications.

Scudder, H. E. (1886). The Bostonians, by Henry James. *The Atlantic Monthly.* Retrieved from https://www.theatlantic.com/past/docs/unbound/classrev/the bosto.htm

Shapere, D. (1982). The concept of observation in science and philosophy. *Philosophy of Science, 49*(4), 485–525.

Simonton, D. K. (2004). *Creativity in science: Chance, logic, genius, and zeitgeist.* Cambridge: Cambridge University Press.

Skinner, B. F. (1938). *The behavior of organisms.* New York: Appleton-Century-Crofts.

Skinner, B. F. (1953). *Science and human behavior*. New York: Simon & Schuster.

Smith, L. D. (1990). Metaphors of knowledge and behavior in the behaviorist tradition. In D. Leary (ed.), *Metaphors in the history of psychology* (pp. 239–265). New York: Cambridge University Press.

Smythe, W. E. (ed.). (1998). *Toward a psychology of persons*. New York: Erlbaum.

Staats, A. W. (1991). Unified positivism and unification psychology: Fad or new field? *American Psychologist*, 46(9), 899–912.

Staats, A. W. (1999). Unifying psychology requires new infrastructure, theory, method, and a research agenda. *Review of General Psychology*, 3, 3–13.

Stafford, B. M. (2001). *Visual analogy: Consciousness as the art of connecting*. Cambridge: MIT Press.

Stam, H. (1998). The dispersal of subjectivity and the problem of persons in psychology. In W. Smythe (ed.), *Toward a psychology of persons* (pp. 221–244). New York: Erlbaum.

Stein, E. (1964). *On the problem of empathy*. W. Stein, trans. Dordrecht: Springer Science and Business. Originally published 1917.

Stroebe, W., & Strack, F. (2014). The alleged crisis and the illusion of exact replication. *Perspectives on Psychological Science*, 9(1), 59–71.

Stuart, M. (2018). How thought experiments increase understanding. In Michael T. Stuart, Yiftach J. H. Fehige, & James Robert Brown (eds.), *The Routledge companion to thought experiments* (pp. 526–544). London: Routledge.

Sundararajan, L. (2015). Indigenous psychology: Grounding science in culture, why and how? *Journal for the Theory of Social Behaviour*, 45(1), 64–81.

Teo, T. (2015). Critical psychology: A geography of intellectual engagement and resistance. *American Psychologist*, 70(3), 243–254.

Teo, T. (2017a). From psychological science to the psychological humanities: Building a general theory of subjectivity. *Review of General Psychology*, 21(4), 281–291.

Teo, T. (2017b, March). The epistemic, practical, and emancipatory interests of the psychological humanities in theoretical refection. In T. Teo (Chair), *Reenvisioning theoretical psychology: Rebels with(out) a cause?* Symposium (Presidential Forum) conducted at the Midwinter Meeting of the Society for Theoretical and Philosophical Psychology, Richmond, VA.

Teo, T. (2018).The role of values, power, and money in the psydisciplines. In *Outline of theoretical psychology: Palgrave studies in the theory and history of psychology* (pp. 179–199). London: Palgrave Macmillan.

Thagard, P. (2014). Creative intuition: How EUREKA results from three neural mechanisms. In L. Osbeck & B. Held (eds.), *Rational intuition: Philosophical roots, scientific investigations* (pp. 287–306). New York: Cambridge University Press.

Thorndike, R. L., & Hagen, E. P. (1969). *Measurement and evaluation in psychology and education*. New York: John Wiley & Sons.

Tissaw, M. A., & Osbeck, L. M. (2007). On critical engagement with the mainstream: Introduction. *Theory & Psychology*, 17(2), 155–168.

Titchener, E. B. (1899). Structural and functional psychology. *Philosophical Review*, 8, 290–299.

Titchener, E. B. (1912). The schema of introspection. *American Journal of Psychology*, 23, 485–508.

Tjeltveit, A. (1999). *Ethics and values in psychotherapy*. London: Routledge.

Tolman, E. C. (1948). Cognitive maps in rats and men. *Psychological Review*, 55(4), 189–208.

Toon, A. (2012). *Models as make-believe: Imagination, fiction and scientific representation*. London: Palgrave Macmillan.

Tweney, R. D. (1985). Faraday's discovery of induction: A cognitive approach. In D. Gooding (ed.), *Faraday rediscovered* (pp. 189–209). London: Palgrave.

Varela, F. J., Thompson, E., & Rosch, E. (2017). *The embodied mind: Cognitive science and human experience*. Cambridge: MIT Press. Originally published 1991.

Vescio, B. (2003). Introduction. In W. James, *Pragmatism: A new name for some old ways of thinking* (pp. ix–xiiii) New York: Barnes & Noble.

Vosniadou, S., & Ortony, A. (eds.). (1989). *Similarity and analogical reasoning*. New York: Cambridge University Press.

Vygotsky, L. S. (1978). *Mind in society: The development of higher mental process*. M. Cole, trans. Cambridge: Harvard University Press.

Wagenknecht, S., Nersessian, N. J., & Andersen, H. (eds.). (2015). *Empirical philosophy of science: Introducing qualitative methods into philosophy of science*. Cham: Springer International.

Watson, J. B. (1913). Psychology as the behaviorist views it. *Psychological Review*, 20 (2), 158–177.

Weber, M. (1946). In H. H. Gerth & C. Wright Mills (trans. and ed.), *Max Weber: Essays in Sociology* (pp. 129–156). New York: Oxford University Press.

Weick, K. E. (1995). *Sensemaking in organizations*. Thousand Oaks: SAGE.

Weinfurt, K. (2003). Book review: *Experience, grammar, and the stuff of persons*. *Theory & Psychology*, 15(3), 407–409.

Wertheimer, M. (1981). Einstein: The thinking that led to the theory of relativity. In R. Tweney, M. Doherty, & C. Mynatt (eds.), *On scientific thinking* (pp. 192–211). New York: Columbia University Press.

Wertz, F. J. (2014). Qualitative inquiry in the history of psychology. *Qualitative Psychology*, 1(1), 4–16.

Wertz, F. J. (2016). Outline of the relationship among transcendental phenomenology, phenomenological psychology, and the sciences of persons. *Schutzian Research: A Yearbook in Lifeworldly Phenomenology and Qualitative Social Sciences*, 8, 139–162.

Wertz, F. J., Charmaz, K., McMullen, L. M., Josselson, R., Anderson, R., & McSpadden, E. (2011). *Five ways of doing qualitative analysis*. New York: Guilford.

Wheelwright, P. (1962). *Metaphor and reality*. Bloomington: Indiana University Press.

Whewell, W. (1844). *The philosophy of the inductive sciences* (2 vols., 2nd ed.). London: J. W. Parker.

Williams, R., & Robinson, D. (2015). *Scientism: The new orthodoxy*. Sydney: Bloomsbury Academic.

Wittgenstein, L. (1953). *Philosophical investigations*. G. E. M. Anscombe, trans. Oxford: Blackwell.

Woolhouse, C. (2017). Multimodal life history narrative. *Narrative Inquiry,* 27(1), 109–131.

Wundt, W. (1882). *Die Aufgaben der experimentellen psychologie. Unsere Zeit,* 18, 389–406.

Zachar, P. (2014). *A metaphysics of psychopathology.* Cambridge: MIT Press.

INDEX

acting person framework, 2, 4, 10, 40, 46, 125
  art and, 110–111
  imaginative sense-making and, 80
  James brothers and, 112, 125
  scientist as, 8
activities, 39–40
aesthetic values, 19, 123
agency, 9, 108, 110
analogy, 70–78
  Hadamard on, 75–77
  imagination and visualization and, 74–78
  metaphor as analogical models, 70–72
  Poincaré and, 70–72
  scientific reasoning through, 77–78
Angell, J. R., 21
Araujo, S. F., 43–44
Aristotle, 4, 54, 69

Bacon, F., 43, 48, 51–52, 53, 54, 57
Beller, S., 105
Bender, A., 105
Bentley, M., 26
bioengineering, 6, 7, 78, 81
Black, Max, 69
Bonnet, Charles, 56
Bostonians, The (James, 2000/1886), 113–115
Bowne, Borden P., 5
Bridgman, P., ix
Bronowski, J., 123
Bruner, Jerome, 66–68, 69, 70–71, 78, 90, 108
  emotional experience and, 76

case analysis, 18, 56, 58, 87
categorizational thought, 66–67
Chalmers, A., 28
Chandrasekharen, Sanjay, 6
cognitive diversity, 105
cognitive map, 63–66

Cognitive Maps in Rats and Men (Tolman, 1948), 63–66
cognitive-cultural system, 89, 91
conceptual change and analogy, 62–66
  cognitive map example, 63–66
constructionism, 15, 61, 85, 98, 102, 108
continuity of science, 17, 19, 22–23, 124
Copernicus, Nicolaus, 47
Coplan, A., 103
creative cognition, 66–68
Cronbach, L. J., 14, 30

Danziger, K., 44–46
Darwin, Charles, 70
Daston, L., 55, 56–57, 79–80
Dewey, J., 4, 26, 108
Dilthey, Wilhelm, 14, 103
  disciplinary perspective, 17, 83, 86, 89–90
discontinuity of science, 16–17, 21, 22
Displacement of Concepts (Schön, 1963), 69
divergent cognition, 105
Dosch, H. G., 35–36, 38, 125
Douglas, H., 13, 19

Einfühlung concept, 103
emotion, transactional view of, 26–27
empathy, 8, 103–104
enactivist frameworks, 4–5
epistemic identities, 91, 93, 102
epistemic power, 105
epistemic priorities, 1–2, 6, 9, 10, 11–12, 31, 109, 125–126
  reevaluation of, 36
epistemic values, 11, 19, 21, 24, 28, 31, 33, 35, 91
  consciousness and, 21–22
  moral values and, 22
  observation and, 42
  researcher-as-person model and, 3
evidence, 60–61